CHALLENGES IN CLINICAL PRACTICE

Also by Veronica Bishop:

*Clinical Supervision in Practice: Some Questions, Answers and Guidelines**

Working towards a Research Degree

* Also published by Palgrave

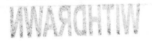

Challenges in Clinical Practice

Professional developments in nursing

Edited by

Veronica Bishop
and
Irene Scott

palgrave

First published 2001 by
PALGRAVE
Houndmills, Basingstoke, Hampshire RG21 6XS and
175 Fifth Avenue, New York, N. Y. 10010
Companies and representatives throughout the world

PALGRAVE is the new global academic imprint of
St. Martin's Press LLC Scholarly and Reference Division and
Palgrave Publishers Ltd (formerly Macmillan Press Ltd).

ISBN 0–333–80231–4 paperback

This book is printed on paper suitable for recycling and
made from fully managed and sustained forest sources.

A catalogue record for this book is available
from the British Library.

Editing and origination by
Aardvark Editorial, Mendham, Suffolk

10   9   8   7   6   5   4   3   2   1
10   09 08 07 06 05 04 03 02 01

Printed and bound in Great Britain by
Creative Print & Design (Wales), Ebbw Vale

Contents

List of Figures and Tables

Figures

Table

List of Boxes

Notes on the Contributors

Denis Anthony RMN RGN RN(Canada) BA(Hons) MSc PhD

Denis is Professor of Nursing Informatics at De Montfort University, Leicester, and since 1984 has maintained an interest in tissue viability, concentrating on risk assessment. He has designed an online course in tissue viability, and experience in related areas has equipped him to create the world's first nursing WWW system. He works closely with health informatics specialists in The Open University and the University of Sheffield and is an advisor in areas as disparate as forensic psychiatric nursing, intensive care nursing workload, pre-hospital treatment and falls in the elderly. Denis is a reviewer for peer journals, and statistical advisor on the editorial board of *Clinical Effectiveness in Nursing*. He is also co-ordinator and chair of the British Computer Society Nursing Special Interest Group/Education Focus Group.

Veronica Bishop PhD MPhil RGN FRSA

Veronica was a late entrant into nursing, having worked in various occupations before qualifying as SRN in 1972. She specialised in intensive care and cardiothoracic nursing before taking up post as a research sister in the Research Department of Anaesthetics at the Royal College of Surgeons, England. Here she obtained her MPhil and PhD while working in a multi-disciplinary clinical research team. Veronica then joined the Civil Service as a nursing officer, where she had responsibility for a large body of research specifically related to nursing and midwifery. In 1992 she moved into the Nursing Directorate in the NHS Executive, with the particular remit to develop nursing practice, and took the national lead on clinical supervision. She is currently Professor of Nursing at De Montfort University and editor of *Nursing Times Research*, a bi-monthly peer review journal for research in the nursing and midwifery professions.

Rebecca Broughton RGN

Rebecca, who has been a registered nurse for 20 years, is currently working as Clinical Effectiveness Co-ordinator at the Leicester Royal Infirmary, University Hospitals of Leicester NHS Trust. Her present role encompasses all aspects of clinical audit and evidence-based practice, and her clinical background has enabled her to ensure that any audit or effectiveness projects are clinically relevant and lead to improvements in patient care.

Dawn Freshwater PhD BA(Hons) RN

At the time of writing Dawn was a senior research fellow in nursing and therapies, a joint appointment with the Mary Seacole Research Centre, De Montfort University, Leicester, and the Department of Nursing, Leicester Royal Infirmary. She was awarded the Sigma Theta Tau for her unique contribution to nursing, and is a community leader in Sigma Theta Tau, the international honour society. Dawn sits on the board of directors of the International Association for Human Caring, is an editorial board member and has co-edited and authored a number of publications. Dawn holds visiting lectureships in North America and has presented at numerous international conferences. She is now Course Director at the Faculty of Medicine, School of Nursing, University of Nottingham.

Jeanette Higginson BMedSci(Hons) RGN

Jeanette qualified as a registered general nurse in 1998 at Sheffield University. She is currently employed as a staff nurse at the Renal and Transplantation Unit, Nottingham City Hospital, where she continues to further her studies in renal nursing.

Irene Scott MSc RGN

Irene trained as a nurse in Manchester and specialised in rehabilitation. After seven years as a Ward Manager, she moved into nursing and in 1996 was appointed Director of Nursing at the Christie Hospital in Manchester. In 1994 Irene joined the executive team at the Leicester Royal Infirmary NHS Trust, which was to be one of two pilot sites for re-engineering. This career move generated particular interest in organisational change and effective leadership. She has contributed to many national debates on clinical governance and the development of care pathways, using a process approach to care. From 1991–97 Irene was co-editor of the *Journal of Cancer Care*, and in 1997 she obtained a Master's degree in Health-care Policy and Organisation. In 1997, in recognition of her contribution to the nursing profession, Irene was made a Visiting Professor of Nursing at De Montfort University, Leicester. Currently Irene is Regional Director of Nursing and Workforce Development at the NHS Executive West Midlands and Honorary Professor at Wolverhampton University.

Tom Tait MA FRSH RNLD RCNT RNT MHSM CertEd

Tom is Senior Lecturer, School of Nursing and Midwifery, De Montfort University, Leicester. He has a wealth and depth of experience in the care of people with learning disabilities. Currently, he is completing his PhD studies in quality of life and its relationship to the care of people with learning disabilities. He is a member of the Royal College of Nursing's national policy and practice forum for learning disability nursing, and has written extensively on his subject.

Foreword

Nurses, midwives and health visitors are entering a period of unprecedented influence and opportunity. The political, social and economic context is such that nurses are in an ideal position to take up the challenges set before them in the National Health Service Plan – fast and convenient care delivered to a consistently high standard, with services available when people require them and tailored to their individual needs.

This excellent book provides a useful tool kit for nurses, midwives and health visitors in engaging in these key themes. Above all, it interprets policy in its relevance to practice, placing practice firmly at the heart of modern nursing.

Paradoxically, change is the one certain element of our lives today. How we deal with that change will determine the place that nurses take in the future NHS. Change is complex, it is unsettling, and it is sometimes frightening – but it also brings opportunities for nurses to influence policy, opportunities to improve care and opportunities to put the patient at the centre of our care systems. Nurses need to understand the process of change and their own behaviour towards it in order to make the most of emerging opportunities.

In reaching a better understanding of the 'power' integral to patient–nurse relationships, the nurse is in a much stronger position to understand change. We all work in partnerships, but, by exploring the true nature of partnership – the give and take, the deals and trade-offs, the potential synergy of joint working – we can better achieve change for our patients.

Clinical governance is a real opportunity for nurses and all our clinical colleagues. Clinical governance – the drive continually to improve patient care – is as much about the way we work as about what we do and how we do it. In order to embrace clinical governance in a meaningful way, the culture of the NHS must change. Openness, accountability with responsibility, learning from each other, acknowledging our mistakes and learning from them, researching and agreeing evidence-based practice – all these must become the norm rather than the exception. Clinical governance must recognise teamworking. Nurses must work with their clinical colleagues, managers and support staff in improving care.

In order for nurses to develop practice and to improve quality, it goes without saying that they need to stay abreast of the latest developments in healthcare, refreshing and renewing their skills and knowledge. We all develop in different ways, at different stages of our lives, which is why the concept of lifelong learning is so critical to today's world. The desire to learn by reflection – to examine our own practice with our peers, to explore the complexities and ambiguities of practice – makes clinical supervision an important personal and organisational developmental tool.

Nursing has some wonderful examples of clinical practice development. As I visit hospitals and primary care settings in the NHS, I am constantly enthused by the variety, depth and breadth of the practice that my colleagues are pursuing. But this is still too patchy. The ability of nurses to develop practice seems still to depend too much on individual enthusiasm rather than organisational commitment. It is sad that some of the best practice development sites falter after the lead individual departs. By exploring the barriers and obstacles, as well as by discovering the factors that facilitate and enable practice to develop, we can better find a way ahead 'to liberate the talents of all'.

Last, but not least, the authors explore the role of informatics and IT in nursing practice. These applications must be to the benefit of the patient. For too long in the NHS, IT systems were more about business efficiency than patient care. I am delighted that this attitude is now well in the past. NHS Direct, for example, is a nurse-led, innovative decision support system enabling patients to get fast, accurate and responsive advice as and when they want it. Nurses, midwives and health visitors must be at the forefront of forthcoming developments.

I welcome this book and feel sure that it will become a standard for nurses, midwives and health visitors who want to explore their practice and develop as people. Congratulations to the editors, Veronica Bishop and Irene Scott, and to the chapter authors, for this excellent contribution.

SARAH MULLALLY
Chief Nursing Officer/Director of Nursing

Acknowledgements

The authors and publishers thank HMSO for permission to reproduce Figure 2.2 from *A First Class Service: Quality in the New NHS* (DoH, 1998, p. 8). Crown copyright material is reproduced with the permission of the Controller of Her Majesty's Stationery Office.

Every effort has been made to trace all the copyright holders but if any have been inadvertently overlooked the publishers will be pleased to make the necessary arrangements at the first opportunity.

List of Abbreviations

CPHVA	Community Practitioners and Health Visitors Association
CRD	Centre for Reviews and Dissemination
DoH	Department of Health
HIMP	Health Improvement Programme
HISS	hospital information support system
HSF	Health Service Framework
IT	information technology
LAN	local area network
NDU	nursing development unit
NHS	National Health Service
NHSE	National Health Service Executive
NHSME	National Health Service Management Executive
NICE	National Institute for Clinical Excellence
NSF	National Service Framework
PC	personal computer
R&D	research and development
RCN	Royal College of Nursing
ScHARR	School of Health and Related Research
UKCC	United Kingdom Central Council
URL	uniform resource locator
WP	word processor
WWW	World Wide Web

Introduction

An Overview of Current Changes in the NHS in Relation to Nursing

Veronica Bishop and Irene Scott

The aim of this chapter is to introduce the reader to current changes in the National Health Service (NHS) in relation to nursing and to highlight key issues which are further developed in the following chapters. Constant changes in politics and ever-increasing advances in technology have combined to present a greater challenge than ever in meeting the demands of the UK population, which in turn has ever-increasing expectations. The role of evidence-based practice, clinical governance and clinical supervision, as well as research and development in nursing, in terms of the profession's ability to deliver knowledgeable care, is discussed, the need for support for practitioners being stressed.

Organisational changes in the NHS over the past 20 years

There have been successive changes in the organisation of the NHS over the past 20 years, stemming from the Thatcher government's determination to wrest control of the service from doctors, and from the need to meet the many challenges that Europe's largest employing organisation faces. A major reorganisation during this period of change related to the service's funding mechanisms. Government monies previously distributed via regions to Health Authorities to fund systems of care were then

allocated via a commercially styled operation that split the supply
and provision functions of healthcare by developing an 'internal'
market. This system, adapted from the American insurance
system, created in the UK an 'internal market' within the health
services, which had the possible advantage of a more competi-
tive and cost-conscious system, with the attendant disadvantage
of an account-style mentality (and bureaucracy) over-riding the
needs of the population. The drive to contain or 'ration' healthcare was eventually to fall to GPs, who became, often with great
reluctance, fundholders. In other words, the money for care was
awarded to the GP on a weighted per capitatation basis.

The NHS is a major weapon in any political party, and the
recent change of government from Conservative to Labour has
brought changes in service organisation that are still, at the time
of writing, in their developmental stage. Health Authorities, with
a remit to fund appropriate care for their populations (rather
than systems of care as in previous decades), the authorities being
made up of lay people, doctors and other healthcare personnel,
are to take over the purchasing role within regions. GP fund-
holding has ceased and is being replaced with Primary Care
Trusts which, while GP led, will provide local populations with
a wider perspective in the ongoing resource versus needs debate.
As technology advances, and the public becomes more aware
and more educated, with consequently higher expectations, the
debate on the cost-effective use of resources will continue.

The debate is one not only of electoral politics, but also of
power bases, and this book aims to arm nurses in their empowerment in order that they may reach their potential as key players
in the healthcare system and contribute fully to future developments. Nurses must recognise that it is not only in the gift of
politicians to shape the NHS. It has always been, and will continue
to be, the responsibility of those professionals working within it
to assist in the shaping of the service and to create opportunities to influence both local and national policy.

Other changes over the past 20 years that have particularly
impacted on nursing have been the reduction in junior doctors'
hours (DoH, 1991) and the imperative to have a primary care-
led NHS (NHS and Community Care Act 1990). These are
changes that have had a significant impact on acute sector and
community-based staff, and have presented opportunities to

consider new ways of working. Added to this rapidly changing NHS scenario is the fact that the 'user' of the NHS has, quite rightly, become very much at the centre of focus. This culture of change may leave those who are busy trying to get on with their job, of taking care of too many patients, in too little time and with too few resources, emotionally flattened. This need not be the case; indeed, it should not be the case. Rather, it is an opportunity to embrace new ideas and create what Scott (1999) calls a 'let's have a go' mentality; in her view, the key to success in change is excellence in leadership at both clinical and managerial levels.

Changing health needs and patterns of care offer unique opportunities, opportunities for the nurse–patient interface to become stronger and less fragmented, for the nurse to offer care that is sensitive to the cultural needs of patients, to really make care 'user centred'. Opportunities abound within the newly developing frameworks of care for health promotion and health education to come to the fore, an undervalued aspect of nursing that to date has perhaps only really been taken forward by health visitors.

The role and position of nurses and nursing in the development of healthcare today has never been more challenging, but with this challenge comes the moment to be grasped. Never have nurses been presented with such an opportunity to affect the agenda and shape the future of the profession, organisational design and local and national policy. With this opportunity, however, also come many challenges. It is essential that nurses, as professionals, rise to these challenges and exert their expertise, which is unique in healthcare provision.

The uniqueness of this professional group is grounded in its closeness to the very essence of an individual's healthcare experience. The breadth and depth of nursing demonstrate that all aspects of other healthcarers' roles implicate the nurse in a holistic manner. While treatment and diagnosis are principally the remit of the medical profession, it is the nurse who measures, monitors, manages and designs the delivery of care over a 24-hour period throughout the care need of an episode of ill health. Likewise, it is the nurse who designs, delivers and monitors the effectiveness of health education at every point of a person's growth.

This book aims to assist in this challenge, drawing on the current agenda and supporting nurses in addressing the critical challenges of the current era. Given the speed of change and the need for nurses to be responsive to these changes, indeed sometimes to bring about these changes, this publication must clearly be quite focused in achieving its aims of supporting the nurses involved in change. For this reason, we have selected high-profile agenda issues of the day, with the aim of demystifying them, and we aim to provide some practical and proven solutions to achieving change.

Thinking the unthinkable

To rise to the challenges of today's healthcare agenda, it is essential to understand and recognise the need for excellence in change management, Chapter 1 providing an insight into the facilitators and inhibitors of this change management. Scott aims to enable the would-be change agent to recognise the need to look back in order to look forward. It is essential to learn from the past in order to enable success to accrue in the future. The retrospectorscope can be an invaluable instrument if properly used rather than mourned over.

It is no longer satisfactory to assume that someone else is going to do it and the rest will follow. The very nature of good change management, which produces sustainable change, relies on shared values, shared goals and therefore shared success. It is necessary then that nurses should aim to have shared skills, not only of a clinical nature, but also in change management. Clearly, not everyone will wish to lead a change management process, but at some time everyone will be affected by and participate in one. It is intended that this book should be of benefit to all professions, but its principal aim is to enable and assist nursing and its related professions in accessing and succeeding in the challenges facing them in today's healthcare system.

The nursing profession has not enjoyed the ability to influence changes in national policy in the same way as has the medical profession. With the passage of time and the growth of many supporting professions, the power base of the medical profession can be seen to be diluting. Now is the time for nurses to rise to this challenge and really make a difference; the profession has a real opportunity to demonstrate an ability to control and manage its own development and indeed the future of the NHS. The clinical governance initiative is seen by many nurse leaders as a unique chance for nurses to grasp their rightful place at the policy and clinical decision-making tables. In Chapter 2, Scott, a leading proponent of clinical governance, explains why this is so and suggests how best to grasp the opportunity.

Autonomy and responsibility

Never have nurses had more scope, such a breadth of areas in which to work or as much possibility for support. There are several driving forces for this, perhaps the most influential being the publication of the United Kingdom Central Council (UKCC) *Scope of Professional Practice* (1992a). The UKCC published this document in 1992 with the aim of providing the nursing and midwifery professions with the means of developing responsive and flexible healthcare services. The impact of *Scope* on practitioners has been substantial (Jowett et al., 1999), with practitioners exploring the principles of *Scope* and what their potential might be within this. Undertaking new roles and crossing traditional barriers requires nurses to demonstrate their competence and accountability; with autonomy comes responsibility, a view shared by Hancock (1997), which is further discussed in the recently published document *Fitness for Practice* (UKCC, 1999a).

Much of the success of any individual will depend on the vision and support of good management and careful career planning. What has improved enormously is the determined inclusion of clinical practice into career advancement in nursing, demonstrated by the introduction of nurse consultant posts, after decades of structures that gave the highest prestige first to educationalists and then to managers. *Making a Difference* (DoH, 1999a) provides an important platform to help the nursing professions to pursue a radical and progressive agenda (Moores, 1999). Drawn from extensive consultation across the profession and related disciplines, it pulls together the aspirations of nursing within the context of the new healthcare agenda and signals the importance of clinical governance, clinical supervision and research-based practice.

Staffing in the NHS: supporting new roles

In considering the role of healthcare delivery for the present and for the future, the agenda must be set in the context of resources, needs and knowledge. At the onset of the new millennium, the NHS has a staffing crisis (DoH, 1999) and is facing the worst shortage of qualified nurses in 25 years (RCN, 1998), with 80 per cent of Trusts experiencing problems with the recruitment of professional staff (Light, 1999). Traditional systems for the provision of healthcare are unable to meet the demands of this scenario, a fact well recognised by most leaders in the NHS and by policy-makers in the Department of Health (DoH). This shared recognition can, however, sometimes seek resolution in different ways, to the confusion of the practitioner in the clinical setting.

There has been a significant increase in the development of nurse-led services, partly because of the reduction in junior doctors' hours (DoH, 1991, 1993b) and partly to move from the existing models of care, which are medically focused, in order to provide care that is more patient centred, more responsive to the clients' specific needs. There are many innovations today that are either now well established or are, with the current ethos of collaborative partnerships, breaking across old barriers. A few examples that come to mind are the newly developed specialist roles, such as nurse-led, instead of medically led, clinics, the collaboration of nurses with the police to develop nurse-led assessment services during arrests, outreach services for the socially excluded, NHS Direct (a nurse-led health helpline), nurse-led walk-in centres and many others besides.

These developments owe much to the work of Pearson (1989) and his colleagues and later to the Sainsbury Family Trust's funding of four nursing developments units (NDUs) based on the philosophy of Pearson and like-minded colleagues. A platform has certainly developed that has encouraged a collaboration between higher education and clinical areas, and in an important paper by Read (1999), attention has been drawn to the importance of proper management planning and support, which are needed to underpin the provision of nurse-led services.

That practitioners move from post to post, and develop their learning and expertise in an individual way tailored to meet their lifestyle and opportunities, is recognised and accepted by the Commission for Education formed by the UKCC in their recently published report *Fitness for Practice* (UKCC, 1999a). Importantly, the report recommends and supports the formalisation of clinical supervision (see recommendation 20). While the recommendations of this report have no professional or legal status at the time of writing, the implications in terms of personal commitment and organisational funding are substantial. In Chapter 3, Bishop, who had the national lead in initiating clinical supervision in the 1990s, discusses why, in her view, clinical supervision will fail without this joint commitment, and clinical practice fail with it (Bishop, 1998).

Clinical practice: the linchpin of professional nursing

Clinical practice is fundamental to nursing, whatever other roles nurses may take on. The power of nursing lies in its ability to provide knowledgeable care and to use that knowledge to bring a quality dimension to a period of a patient or client's life that would be unlikely to be provided by a lay person. Contrary to the impression to be gained from some of the nursing literature, caring is not the prerogative of nurses: there are many people who can and do care. Nursing should be identified by the provision of knowledgeable care. There is a view that:

> nursing must now face the reality that past professional strategies have denied it the power base in clinical practice it now requires to promote leaders who will remain in nursing practice and to have its voice heard in the clinical decision-making process. (Kyzer, 1992, pp. 112–19)

At the beginning of a new era, and a new millennium, nursing has the opportunity, not least through the recently published DoH paper *Making a Difference* (1999a), to play a significant role in healthcare strategies. This opportunity raises issues of professional development, career planning and innovative practices, which are discussed more fully in Chapter 4.

Bringing research into care

Nursing care may be very specific, as performed by specialist nurses such as dialysis nurses, or intravenous therapy nurses. Much of general nursing practice is, however, very diffuse, and to identify single interventions and judge their effectiveness is very difficult with existing measuring instruments. There are so many other variables that cannot be controlled, such as the overall environment, other staff, family and so on. Even where methods of measurement have been devised, finding evidence for sound clinical decisions is not always as easy as it should be. There is not, as yet, sufficient infrastructure to support either well-constructed or well-conducted research in nursing, possibly owing to an inherent lack of understanding of the requirements in terms of resources and expertise. It is neither realistic nor necessary that all qualified nurses should undertake research, but it is a fundamental requirement that they should be able to access and understand research findings.

Chapter 3 offers an insight into bridging the gap between practice and theory, day-to-day care and research-based findings. The phrase 'evidence based' is increasingly entering the discourse surrounding clinical effectiveness in nursing (Bonnell, 1999; Closs and Cheater, 1999). In addition, it was recently reported that 67 per cent of current nursing research is subsidised by the nurses themselves (Hancock, 2000), undoubtedly an indication of the tremendous appetite that nurses have for research knowledge. Why then is it so difficult to get research findings into practice? What are the barriers to the successful implementation of evidence-based nursing practice?

Chapter 3 considers one of the biggest challenges facing nursing, that of how to ensure that nursing care is founded upon the best available evidence – in other words to how to get research into practice. It is, however, imperative to the future of nursing as an emerging profession that this is achieved by accountable and professional means. The care that patients receive is dependent upon a number of factors, not least the education and the training that nurses and midwives receive. Freshwater and Broughton argue that, in order to ensure that nursing practice is substantiated by the best available evidence, it is necessary to improve the capability of nurses and midwives to seek out and achieve ownership of the appropriate evidence.

Demonstrating their belief in nurses and nursing, the authors of Chapter 5 have drawn nurses into the debate, used their collective and personal experiences, and supported much of the discussion with reference to highly respected authors and researchers in both nursing and other areas of healthcare. The text is designed not in a prescriptive manner but in such a way as to provide an opportunity for debate and flexibility, as well as food for thought, which may be translated by readers into a context that will stimulate thinking relevant to their area of practice and their current area of challenge.

Cultural challenges: involving carers and utilising IT

While there are many nurses who have, as a matter of course, sought to involve patients' carers, this is not the norm. Although there is a strong government drive to change this, demonstrated by the demand for the involvement of service users, and the heavy focus on the study of carers in DoH-funded projects, there is a long way to go in changing the healthcare culture from one that is essentially paternalistic to one that shares its power base. We need to reconsider the role of nursing not only within the healthcare team, and at the clinical table, but also at the power shift in our relationship with patients and careers.

Nursing accounts for approximately 80 per cent of the direct care that patients receive, which often involves personal and intimate care activities. Nurses are therefore in a unique situation to develop therapeutic, complex relationships with their patients. Within these relationships, there is a hidden danger that nursing staff may, unintentionally, establish an unequal power system and remain ignorant of how this can impact upon those for whom they care. Contemporary healthcare demands an approach that is underpinned by productive partnerships between nursing staff and those in their care. The development of a nurse–patient or nurse–informal carer partnership where people can make their own healthcare decisions will make a significant contribution to enhancing overall patient care. In Chapter 6, Tom Tait and Jeanette Higginson seek systematically to examine the notion of power in nursing and how it can impact upon the relationships between nurse, informal carer and patient.

Some people love technology; others resist it! The fact of the matter is that it is here to stay, and, approached with a willingness to be open, IT has a great deal to offer. Denis Anthony, in Chapter 7, takes the reader on a clinically based tour of IT, exploring the options currently available. He stresses that nurses in the clinical area should not worry about the technology itself but consider what it might offer to them in their practice. Typical nursing functions that are helped by IT include evidence-based practice and research, continuing education and professional development, planning and executing nursing care, and patient information. This chapter explores the use of IT in nursing practice, concentrating on those aspects of IT that assist the nurse practically.

Tomorrow's world: nursing for the future

Nursing in England has the wind of change behind it (Johnston, 1999a). The reader needs to consider, in the light of recent history, what permutations are likely for skill mix in an economy that is struggling to support an increasingly elderly population and to keep up with the explosion in technology. Will we develop into an all-graduate profession, or will we have a hierarchy that is led by a minority of specialist staff? What will identify the 'expert' nurse, and how best may the profession be represented at the policy table? The leading question should perhaps be 'how can the NHS provide individualised patient care that is user centred and meets the demands of a knowledgeable and litigious society in an economy indicating little sign of expansion?' These are the real challenges of healthcare professionals.

Perhaps the contribution of nurses, who are the largest group of professional staff in the NHS, will be better understood as the configuration of services changes in response to users' and carers' demands, rather than being traditionally/medically driven. Training and education programmes for student nurses are already involving patients and families; ethnic and black minorities are rightly influencing our services to their populations; the socially excluded are at last beginning to be heard. This has a little to do with politics and a great deal to do with the confidence of the nursing profession in embracing such diverse agendas.

The government has committed itself in *Making a Difference* (DoH, 1999a), the national strategy for nursing in England, and has placed research highly in that portfolio. Whatever the national priorities are, it must be a priority of members of the profession to care for the profession, to support each other and to share their undoubted expertise.

Historically, nursing has never appeared to be better placed to take forward a new professional status that will empower its practitioners to provide the care they are well equipped to do and to take their rightful place in society, at the bedside and at the policy table. This will not be achieved by innovation alone, however well publicised. It will only be achieved, in the long term, by nursing continuing to show its reflective and dynamic abilities, and by sound research to underpin its practice. If we support each other and base our knowledge on sound education and research, we can meet any challenge.

Key Point Summary

- Change may be fun!

- Ensure good support systems that challenge you

- Nursing is the key to quality healthcare provision

- Read this book a bit at a time

1

The Management of Change

Irene Scott

'We tried it before and it didn't work!' How often have we heard these words uttered? Have we ever stopped to consider what it is that makes change successful?

The aim of this chapter is to generate a recognition of the complexities of change management and provide the reader with some tools to enable successful and sustainable change. The role of nurses in change management is essential if nursing is to establish a strong position in shaping the future of healthcare, the delivery of care and the development of policy. The chapter discusses and identifies the enablers and inhibitors of change management, all of which should and can be put into the context of both micro and macro change. The power and cultural issues influencing change are discussed and are transposed into a model that provides a step-by-step guide for any would-be change agent. The model is based on a care pathways 'tool kit' designed by a multi-professional/multi-disciplinary team in the Trent region, UK, looking to influence the future of cancer services.

In order to know where we are going and to plan how we are going to get there, we need to understand not only where we are coming from, but also what has influenced the design of where we stand today. We need to be cognisant of lessons learnt and to be able to recognise all the contributing factors, political, socio-logical and humanistic. This chapter aims to draw out the many issues involved in the complexities of change management as well as to highlight the opportunities, levers and inhibitors to be considered. It provides one model for achieving change and offers practical advice for the would-be change leader.

Whatever the change intended, whether in clinical practice, in the design of a complete patient process or indeed in the whole change of an organisation, the principles remain the same. The aim in change management must be to produce sustainable change; how often does one hear people resist change by saying 'We tried it before and it didn't work'? All too often, this comment is generated out of an inability to recognise the real tools and techniques of change management. A cautionary note should be issued at this point. Not all change is successful, and this must be recognised from the start. However, it is better to have tried and learnt from failure than never to have tried at all. All lessons are valuable in shaping the future.

Over the past five decades the NHS has been subjected to many changes in its quest for improving the efficiency and quality of healthcare. There are many texts describing the journey of the NHS through organisational and management change, financial probity (Brindle, 1998; Ham, 1992) and, more recently, outcomes of diagnosis, treatment and care. At the beginning of the 21st century, however, the changes faced by healthcare professionals demand a critical change in thinking.

This requires changing the traditional culture of the NHS, which could easily be described as conservative, in the non-political sense, and restrictive. It is a culture that has been finely tuned and honed, and is passed down from one generation to another. Those new members joining the system can be forgiven for discarding their newly taught thinking accessed through universities in favour of that perpetuated by an older society. Many find it easier to comply with and slip into the old ways of working in order to enable an easy working relationship with established professionals. Consider the newly qualified nurse who has been educated to challenge and question practice. This individual can be seen as both threatening and disrespectful of the ward sister, of long-experienced colleagues, not least of the medical profession and others with whom he or she is required to work. It therefore becomes easier for this individual to adopt old ways of working simply to 'fit in'. The passage of change therefore becomes protracted, inhibited and often laborious.

The newly established expression in healthcare 'language' today is 'clinical governance', a statement that trips off the tongue but is not yet commonly understood. The reason for the array of interpretations lies within the expectations and common practices learned from the predecessors of individual professional groups. Clinical governance is comprehensively covered in Chapter 2, but it must be noted at this early stage that every action of every professional, whether overt or covert, is a matter of the clinical governance agenda. The success of this agenda is dependent upon our ability as professionals to enable and enact change on a continuum. That is, to achieve change we need the tools and the techniques, we need to recognise and understand the inhibitors and the facilitators, and we need to 'think the unthinkable'.

Influence and historical development

To know where we are going, we must understand where we are coming from. This comment is applicable to all change practice and should recognise both the macro and the micro historical influences in the development and design of healthcare. The NHS has a history, as do the individual organisations and professions who serve in it. This history has been influenced by many factors, including political, sociological and humanistic ones.

In considering the political context of the development of the NHS, it should be recognised that it is a service that touches the lives of everyone. Consequently, whatever the political colour and leadership of the day, it makes a very useful political football, one government regime blaming another for its ineffectual or even destructive actions. However, the high profile of the NHS makes any political party strive for success in improving the service. Yet we must recognise that it is not only in the gift of politicians to shape the NHS. It has always been, and will continue to be, the responsibility of those professionals working within it to assist in the shaping of the service and to create the opportunity to influence both local and national policy.

The history of healthcare clearly goes beyond the development of the NHS, but for the purposes of this book, we will start at the point of the development and implementation of the NHS Act in 1946. Any reader wishing to learn about issues leading to the Act is advised to read Ham (1992).

The development and implementation of the NHS is in itself a good example of change management. It is interesting to consider how the Act was designed and what factors were to influence its successful implementation. In essence, the NHS was ultimately founded on what was possible rather than on what was desirable. The main influence on its structure and focus was the medical profession. Indeed, the implementation was made on many concessions for doctors, specifically hospital doctors, Aneurin Bevan, the then Health Minister, being quoted as saying that that he had 'stuffed their mouths with gold' (Abel-Smith, 1964, p. 480 in Ham, 1992, p. 14). An agreement was reached upon many bargaining points, not least the option to retain private practice and the introduction of distinction awards to enhance earning potential. This then set the scene for the power of the medical profession, which, in the view of many (Abel-Smith, 1964; Ham, 1992; Webster, 1988) has held the NHS in check ever since its inception. This power, combined with the position granted to the medical profession by society, makes the medical profession the only profession that holds a statutory right to be consulted on change in the NHS.

The medical profession

The position of doctors in society is easily expounded. The development of the NHS was seen by many as a gift, removing the need to pay at source for healthcare and providing a service that was to be available to all. After the war years (1939–45), the birth of a free health service was seen as a desperately needed benefaction, softening the blows of industrialisation and poor living that many suffered and changing the role of Poor Law hospitals from places of squalor to, what became for many, centres of real expertise. The doctor was central to these changes, being unchallenged in his authority, even by Parliament, a factor that is quickly changing today. In this scenario, the power of this healthcare group was paramount and indeed strengthened with the combined advancement of medical research, political power in academia and the developing Royal Colleges. So the scene is set for the future of change management and the future of healthcare in the UK.

The nursing profession

Having established that the main source of power lies at the heart of the development of the NHS and the influence of the medical profession, what is the position of the nursing profession, which, while having far more members, has held little or no power? The role of the nurse is generated from the care role played by the mother in the family unit and from the early tradition of caring nuns, who practised servitude and humility. Thus the nurse in the hospital was initially seen not as an employee with particular skills but as someone 'below stairs', in a position of servitude to clean and tend to the patients. This very brief potted history illustrates the attitudes affecting the position of the nursing profession today and sets the scene for the status of the nurse in relation to change management and the development of healthcare.

The tradition that nurses were not to question the care or treatment prescribed by doctors but were required to act on the instruction or order has only relatively recently been formally challenged (UKCC, 1992b). This altered position of nursing can clearly be seen to lie with the matriarch of nursing change, Florence Nightingale, who challenged and ultimately changed the relationship between doctor and nurse. It is my opinion that as a result of her actions, nurses became the subordinates of the matron instead of the medical consultant. Thus the nursing hierarchy was born, one which, ironically, mimicked the medical model and which, to a greater or lesser extent, still exists today.

The power of the matron remained within nursing for many years, the role, as with that of the consultant in medicine, being pinnacled by society and therefore able to hold onto its power well into the 1970s, in some notable cases beyond this. Indeed, it is with some irony that, as a nurse trained in the early 1970s, I remember that two of the first things I was taught in my preliminary training school were how to fold a comparatively non-complex nurse's hat and how to curtsy to matron! Despite the speed of the changes, this was a comparatively short time ago. In more recent times in my role as Director of Nursing, I was to learn that the beautifully carved bench that adorned the corridor outside my office was commonly known as the 'naughty bench': attendance at matron's office was expected only as a result of wrong-doing. It is interesting to note that, even at the end of the 20th century, there remained a culture of blame implying that, if a request were made to see an individual, something must be wrong, a belief that took several years to change.

It is interesting that despite the many demonstrable changes and developments in nursing, such as a move to be recognised as a profession, the removal of enrolled nurse training, the move to a greater theory-based education, a plethora of specialisation and not least the development of the auxiliary nursing role, there remains a propensity to hold onto some form of hierarchy in nursing. Clinical grading, for example, although not intended to do so, served to embed even further a hierarchical structure. The nursing profession has clung to its hierarchy model, seeing that society equates position and the concomitant financial reward with power.

Power is the tool by which to make change, and in a society such as the NHS, power is achieved by education and intellect, which is focused in healthcare provision in one of its many aspects. With the advent of nurse training, nurses became the helpers rather than the servants of doctors, a step forward in collaborative working, although nurses were still seen as being subordinate rather than equal. Until the implementation of Project 2000 in 1989, which moved nurse education and training out of hospital schools of nursing and into higher education institutions, nurses were trained in an apprentice-based and somewhat prescriptive manner. Even though Project 2000 has been in place for more than 10 years at the time of writing, nurses educated in this manner still constitute only 20 per cent of all registered nurses, and there is some dissent over the value of a well-qualified nurse workforce.

Nursing continues the struggle to be recognised as a profession, in that a profession holds the distinct right to control its own work and its own development, and while there remains a tension between many of the traditions rooted in nursing and the development of practice based on research and evidence, there will continue to be a debate surrounding the professional status of nursing and nurses.

Administration and management of healthcare

Throughout the history of the NHS, there has been a drive to improve the management of the service. Bringing this down to a very local level, there is the development in hospital management posts, from company secretary status to general manager and latterly to chief executive authority. There have been numerous attempts to reduce management costs to enhance the finance available for patient care, and there have been numerous suggestions on what constitutes a manager. It was not until more recent years that leadership was seen to be an essential element in achieving success, in terms not solely of quantity, but also of quality. The chief executive in today's NHS is held to account for almost all activities in his or her Trust, including the appointment of most senior staff, health and safety, and, more recently, the development of the clinical governance agenda. The power placed upon and held by these individuals is clearly demonstrable.

Perspectives on change

The healthcare organisation is complex in comparison to its industrial counterpart, grappling with numerous agendas and agencies as well as the nation's health. Organisational success is dependent upon the organisational structure, which is in turn influenced by business objectives, rather than the other way around (Audit Commission, 1996; Hammer and Champy, 1993; Kennerfalk and Klefsjø, 1995). It is commonplace today to read of reshaping the organisational structure, which has usually meant 'delayering' or reducing the number of managers. Indeed, the 'New Labour' government, on election in 1997, immediately announced that major savings should be made by reducing management costs (ScHARR, 1997). However, work undertaken by the Institute of Employment in 1995 concluded that 'the most successful did not rely on job cuts alone, but involved the redesign of processes' (Audit Commission, 1996, p. 3). It is clearly important in the design of change to understand how the structure of the organisation affects the work and natural progress. In achieving successful change, the change must be seen by the staff as an improvement, otherwise, because of the culture and inbred traditions, the members will continue to employ the old ways.

Many authors (Hammer and Champy, 1993; Harrison et al., 1992; Kennerfalk and Klefsjø, 1995) suggest that, to achieve sustainable change, the culture of the organisation must change. The organisation may, for our purposes, be a ward, a department or a team in any healthcare setting. Alternatively, the organisation may be viewed as the directorate or whole institution. It is not enough, however, to change the culture of the organisation as culture does not stand alone; it *must* be compatible with the values of the organisation. This would suggest that, in changing an organisation, the values must be realigned, so there is a requirement to agree on and/or change the values of the organisation. Conversely, a change in the values of the organisation should act as a driver for a change in the culture.

Culture as a key influence on change

It is possible that there is no consensus on the definition of culture, but an easy descriptor is captured by 'the way we do things around here', which is a derivative of Hague's (1993, p. 2) sociological definition:

> reflecting how those in it think and act as they carry out their tasks. It shows how we do things here.

The culture of the NHS has developed over the past 50 years and has been transmitted from one generation to another (Harrison et al., 1992), the beliefs and behaviours of the individuals being reinforced as its ideologies, beliefs and rituals are passed down to new members (Ogbonna, 1991). While there is no evidence of a definition of 'health culture', it may be assumed that the structure and resultant actions and beliefs of those within define the orientation of the culture. Indeed, it could be seen that the structure of the organisation is a part of the culture. It is therefore necessary to consider that the greatest challenge to implementing and sustaining change is in bringing about a change in culture. However, the healthcare organisation is complex in the number of constituent professional groups that comprise it. Each professional group will have its own culture, and this will be influenced by both internal and external pressures.

Consider the following:

- Who is in your team or department; whom are you reliant upon to succeed both personally and professionally?
- How are the outcomes of your care delivery going to be influenced by others in your team or department?
- Which professional bodies influence the way in which you work and how your colleagues work?
- Who in your team or department belongs to another team or department and may bring other values with them?

The strengths of the individual cultures will play a central role in determining the culture as a whole (Harrison et al., 1992). This would suggest that the dominant culture may determine how quickly, or even whether, the organisation will change.

Inhibitors of change: power and accountability

We have ascertained that the success of organisational change is dependent upon a cohesiveness of the key players and a realignment of the culture with the values of the organisation. We must, however, also identify the influence of power, which must not be underestimated in achieving real success. In essence, it may be argued that power and culture go hand in hand.

The organisation of healthcare as we know it today has been developed around the medical profession, other health professionals supporting medical activity. Power may be described on two levels, micro and macro (Harrison et al., 1992). The macro power may be determined as the role adopted by external bodies such as the Royal Colleges. These august bodies have played a major part in influencing government policy and have secured the right to be consulted on all manner of changes, a right now beginning to be exerted by nursing's Royal College.

Micro power can be seen as the power exerted by individuals at a local level, the dominant ward sister or the consultant doctors within the team. Indeed, the latter have a level of power not yet enjoyed by most in that they control the work flows, diagnosis and treatment. While it may be inappropriate for those not medically qualified to challenge diagnosis and treatment, work flow has become a sharp focus for the managers of healthcare in determining how hospital finances are spent.

It must be recognised that power is not now owned solely by the medical profession, but may also be positioned in the hierarchy of the organisations. It is interesting to consider why the nursing profession has clung to its hierarchy. It may be argued that one of the greatest challenges in achieving successful change in nursing is to flatten the hierarchy, but, in considering this, one must identify what purpose it currently serves and how this may be met within a new culture. Change on its own is certainly disruptive and unsettling, and may defeat the overall purpose of this particular change – to improve nurses' contribution to healthcare services. To avoid this, the discussion points in this chapter need to be considered.

Power may also be seen in individual professional groups or indeed in individual teams, recognising that two individuals may constitute a team. Individual groups may express power when there are conflicts of objectives and interests, indicating that values must be shared when aiming to achieve successful change. It has been identified in a major change programme that, when changing from a function- to a process-based organisation, many middle managers who become 'at risk' of losing their jobs will do anything to undermine both the individuals involved and the change process.

There is no professional group in today's healthcare system that has the sole rights to power in the industry of healthcare. It has been recognised that the behaviours and attitudes of managers to other members of the organisation are essential to achieve change. Historically, leaders have controlled rather than organised, holding their followers in check rather than promoting evolution (Bennis, 1985). Today, we may face the challenge of the 'double whammy' caused by the increasing number of doctors moving into managerial roles. The project leader for the change management project at a major city hospital recognised that, to sustain process development, active and visible leadership was required of the clinical directors, all of whom were doctors. Without this presence of powerful clinical leadership, the projects were seen to be at risk.

Authors of gender and professional issues would argue that much of the power influence of the medical profession is attributed to paternalism as well as to the positioning of the male over the female in society (Davies, 1995). Recognising that the supporting healthcare professions are predominantly female, it could be argued that any change concept in healthcare must first consider the position of the doctor within the change programme. The change must include and employ the participation of the medical profession, otherwise the implementation of change will be weakened or result in failure. It is of course interesting that, as career opportunities for women widen, many medical schools are demonstrating a higher ratio of female to male medical students. Therefore, a review of this paternalistic influence over change would make an interesting study in years to come.

The organisation of healthcare

It could be argued that while the NHS was established for the patients, it was organised around doctors, other professional groups and departmental working. This organisation of care produces protracted, lengthy and often unnecessary relationships with patients as they pass through the NHS system, where they are passed from one professional group to another and from one department to another (Figure 1.1). At no one time is there any healthcare individual who is responsible for, or indeed recognises and understands, the total process of care. The patient is unwittingly treated like a parcel and is unlikely to have much understanding of the reasoning behind the processes to which she or he is subjected. Function and process have outweighed the importance of the person within, the individual.

Process and function: is there a relationship?

In determining how process differs from function, it is essential to consider the work of those authors who have explored both organisational structures and change management. These authors have all considered or developed models of change around a particular set of processes. Processes have always existed in

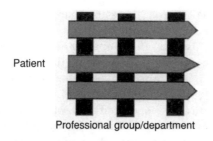

Patient

Professional group/department

Figure 1.1   Patients' travel hindered through
departmental and professional silos

industry and healthcare, even in the most traditional functional
organisations (Hammer, 1993). Process is defined by Hammer
and Champy (1993, p. 35) as:

> a collection of activities that takes one or more kinds of input and
> creates an output that is of value to the customer.

It is interesting that while the literature on healthcare process
discusses the development of process, there are few definitions
to be found. Keill and Johnson (1994, p. 2) describe a healthcare process as:

> a series of actions or operations to achieve an end result

whereas Dr Helen Bevan, the re-engineering project leader at
Leicester Royal Infirmary NHS Trust in 1997, described process as:

> the patient's journey through the hospital.

It is clear that 'process' is not a term normally applied to healthcare in describing organisation design, yet it is easy to locate the
term 'function' in the healthcare literature. It is, however, also
clear that all activities undertaken in a hospital, either clinical or
operational, are a composite of a variety of processes (Keill and
Johnson, 1994). Keill and Johnson determine that functions are
composed of processes, the function being a larger entity, encom-
passing smaller, more manageable components which are
processes. Yet it could be argued that a series of functions forms
the process. This argument is based on the belief that a patient

process is comprised of everything that happens to the patient from admission, or referral, until discharge.

The description used by these authors focuses quite clearly on the contributing functions for a part of the patient's hospital experience rather than the total experience. The case study of a re-engineering project offered through the work of the Leicester Royal Infirmary identified that while healthcare has been designed around functional units, for example X-ray, operating and outpatient departments, the patient passes across the functions in a horizontal fashion. This lateral process is clearly disturbed by the handing-over of responsibility for the patient from one person and department to another (see Figure 1.1 above), resulting in the patient experiencing a virtual process.

The differences between function-oriented organisations and process-oriented organisations have been described by Kennerfalk and Klefsjø (1995, p. 190) as extreme. While they believe that examples of these extremes do not exist, most organisations will lie somewhere between, closer to one extreme than another (Table 1.1).

If healthcare is to adopt the definition of process described by Bevan (1997), there is clearly a requirement, as described by Hammer and Champy (1993), Kennerfalk and Klefsjø (1995) and Smith Blancett and Flarey (1995), to consider the organisational structure as a reflection of the process activities. In a function-oriented organisation, labour has been divided by work activity or speciality, managers and workers focusing on their own means rather than the broader ends of the organisation. Grouping these resources allows and promotes specialisation as well as the efficient management of similarly skilled personnel (Kennerfalk and Klefsjø, 1995). The literature is conclusive in its beliefs that, to achieve a process-oriented organisation, either in industry or in healthcare, process leadership is essential (Hammer and Champy, 1993; Kennerfalk and Klefsjø, 1995; Smith Blancett and Flarey, 1995). This argument is based on a belief that if responsibility and authority are centralised to a few people in the organisation, the coordination of activity is disjointed and restricted to a functional group or department, the result of the work in the functional groups and departments being focused on the end result of that group or department rather than on the end result of complementary and interdependent groups and departments.

Table 1.1 Differences between function- and process-based organisations (adapted from Kennerfalk and Klefsjø, 1995, p. 190)

	Function oriented	Process oriented
Structure	hierarchic bureaucratic task oriented exclusive	flat consensus teams inclusive
Culture	functional incremental change short-term thinking	process step change visionary strategic
Communication	vertical top down	horizontal bottom up and top down
Personnel	narrow competence	broad competence
Products	simple standardised organisation oriented	complex customer focused customer oriented

The redesign of patient care is a process that crosses all functions, departments and professions, and requires the development of process teams (Hammer, 1993; Hammer and Champy, 1993; Smith Blancett and Flarey, 1995). Each process team has a multiple membership, which in healthcare will essentially encompass all occupational groups, for example doctors, nurses, physiotherapists, porters, clerical staff and so on, under the leadership of a process owner. However, for a process team to be effective, there must be a willingness in the organisation to empower the teams to make judgements and take decisions (Hammer and Champy, 1993; Smith Blancett and Flarey, 1995). It is therefore implicit that the corporate body must buy into the process and that all the team members must share a common belief, their values and goals being aligned.

The concern arises with this approach of a healthcare organisation potentially moving from being multi-function based to being a multi-process organisation. This re-orientation has the potential to introduce a different configuration of independent teams trying to improve their own process, without any consideration of the organisation and development of other processes. There is therefore a requirement of the team to recognise, retain and develop an understanding and recognition of the corporate values and direction of the hospital.

It is clear that the implications of introducing process management into a healthcare environment are considerable, most notable being the impact on organisational structure and orientation. Notwithstanding the requirements we have already identified as being essential in implementing change, process development in healthcare must be underpinned by a change in the overall structure of the organisation, which has previously been seen to change only at an administrative/managerial level (Coombes and Green, 1989; Ham, 1992).

Tools and techniques for achieving change

Understanding how to plan the future can be applied to either a micro or a macro process. The aim may be to change a clinical activity, the organisation of delivery of care, the organisation of the ward or department, or the organisation of a whole patient pathway of care. Whatever the change, the variables and the activities will remain the same. The challenge is to understand the component parts, recognise the inhibitors and the enablers, and employ good planning techniques.

In its simplest form, change in practice can be planned and implemented by employing five steps (see also Figure 1.2).

1. Reviewing the current situation – process mapping
2. Developing a picture of the ideal future – visioning and designing
3. Testing and piloting – the trial process
4. Evaluating the options for the future – producing the optimum
5. Implementation – sustained change and continuous improvement

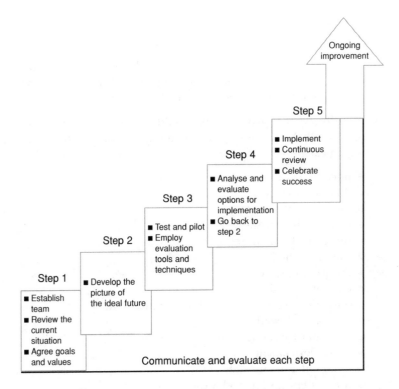

Figure 1.2 Five basic steps to achieving change
(developed by Trent Nurses and Professions Allied to Medicine working group)

Step 1: Process mapping

A description of process mapping was provided by the project
leader in her process redesign work. In the case study, it can be
seen that a series of functions makes up the process. Process
mapping is an exercise to identify all the components, contributions and contributors for an agreed activity. This stage of the
change process is extremely enlightening and enables a close
review of the activity as seen by many individuals, including the
patient. It can also be great fun and is often a catalyst for achieving
a greater understanding in team members and enabling the first
steps in agreeing values and aligning goals. Listed below are the
steps of process mapping.

1. It is clearly important to gain an agreement from the key stakeholders that there is a shared desire to review this activity.

2. Agree what will be included in the change process – for example from the hospital receiving the GP referral to the patient being discharged back to the GP's care.

3. Identify *all* the players. You would, for example, need to involve all the following when aiming to achieve change in a surgical process of care:

   - porters in the post-room
   - theatre porters
   - the medical secretary
   - theatre clinical staff
   - the consultant surgeon
   - the anaesthetist
   - the junior doctor
   - laboratory staff
   - outpatient clinic clerks/administrative staff
   - phlebotomy staff
   - outpatient nursing staff
   - ward clerical staff
   - inpatient nursing staff
   - the patient and/or relatives.

4. Agree a time and a venue for all the representative players to meet. Set aside a substantial amount of time and choose a place that will prevent as much disturbance as possible.

5. Agree the ground rules, for example:

   - everyone has a valuable and equitable contribution
   - if you believe it happens, say it or document it
   - no blaming and shaming
   - don't try and jump to the resolution and the end-stage of the change process.

6. As a large group, agree the high-level process, for example:

   - letter is received from the GP
   - outpatient appointment letter is sent to the patient
   - patient attends for outpatient appointment
   - patient is sent an inpatient appointment

- patient attends for preoperative tests
- patient is admitted
- patient attends theatre for surgery
- inpatient stay
- discharge back to the care of the GP.

The high-level process can, if desired, be divided into two distinct albeit not separate processes:

- Visit = all outpatient attendances
- Stay = period of time spent as an inpatient.

7. Provide each individual with a supply of 'Post-it' notes or sticky-backed paper.

8. Each participant is to write all the activities they perform on the 'Post-it' notes. It is important that only one activity is written on each 'Post-it', so one contributor may have many contributions for inclusion.

9. As a group, and starting with the first step in the process, that is, the receipt of the referral letter, commence the process of sticking each note onto a wall in the sequence in which the events/actions occur. You now have your *process map*.

You will now begin to see the big picture and recognise how complex even the simplest of processes can be.

10. As a group, undertake a detailed analysis of the existing process. When viewing your map, it will now be easy to identify the major activities, the gaps in the service and the unnecessary (non-value adding) activities that hinder and often duplicate what is being done.

11. A detailed analysis can now be undertaken to assess what information is available to support existing practice, what evidence the current process is based upon and what quantitative and qualitative data are available to support practice. This may include local or national guidelines and documentation.

12. Before moving on from this mapping stage, it is essential to ensure an agreement and consensus of the findings, also agreeing to move on to the next step.

Figure 1.3 is taken from work conducted at the Leicester Royal Infirmary NHS Trust during its change programme. The process-mapping exercise demonstrated the unnecessary complexity and prolonged process that the patient experienced following a referral to the hospital for a neurological review. Following critical analysis by the team, they were able to remove all elements of the process that added no value to the determined outcome (non-value-adding steps). The end-product – a single visit clinic (Figure 1.4) – was the consensus of team members.

Step 2: Visioning and designing

At this stage, it is essential to cast aside all barriers and existing limits. Consider an approach that is cased as 'if we had never done this before, how would we do it?' Compare the approach with that of 'zero-based budgeting', used in financial settings (agreeing the total budget depending on the cost of each element). Success at this stage lies in creativity and design, which reflect the needs of the patient rather than the professional or functional needs of the department or organisation. It is essential to enable and develop thinking that is outside the individuals' personal and professional mindset – in other words 'thinking the unthinkable'.

1. Agree what could be achieved, throw aside past experiences and do not be influenced by comments such as 'we tried this before and it didn't work!'

2. Agree what and who will benefit from a change in activity.

3. Identify relevant evidence-based practice and best practice. At this stage, it is useful to access information sources such as the National Institute for Clinical Excellence (NICE), the Cochrane database and the professional bodies.

4. As with Step 1, map out the new process, testing the feasibility and ensuring and articulating the agreement of all the participants.

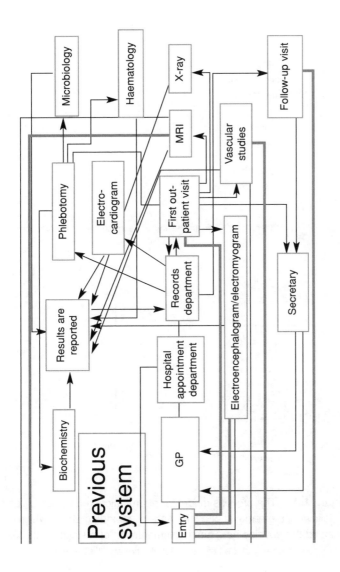

Figure 1.3 The process mapping exercise for a referral for neurological review (courtesy of the Leicester Royal Infirmary NHS Trust)

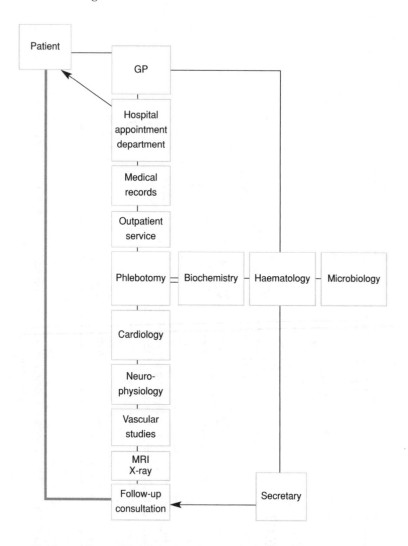

Figure 1.4   The process model for neurological referral as agreed
following the removal of all the non-value-adding steps, which
enabled the development and implementation of a single-visit clinic
(courtesy of the Leicester Royal Infirmary NHS Trust)

Step 3: Testing and piloting the new process

To enable the pilot to run, it is essential to identify what changes in practice are required. One cannot introduce a new way of working over old skills and old processes; it simply will not work. The new process may identify new roles, a new approach to the sharing of skills between the professions or the removal of old activities that may have become traditional, quite simply 'the way we do things around here!'

1. Identify the new skills and competencies required.

2. Identify who is the best person to deliver the skills at the most appropriate time and in the most appropriate place.

3. Agree who needs to be trained to do what, and agree who will deliver the training. (In large-scale change, there is often a need to involve the education institutions to participate and assist in the development of training packages, which can be awarded academic accreditation.)

4. Agree how the new process will be monitored and evaluated and by what means this will happen. This may include an audit of the process, including the patients' experience, clinical outcomes and organisational effectiveness and efficiency. Some simple monitoring techniques are suggested below.

5. Communicate the intentions of the pilot to all who will be affected. It is often useful at this stage to agree a communication plan.

6. Run the pilot for an agreed period of time using a previously determined and agreed sample size.

A few simple monitoring techniques are outlined below.

Patient diaries

It is crucial when making a change to ensure that the user of the service is involved in both the design and evaluation stages of the change process. Patient diaries have been proved to be a useful and enlightening method of collecting data that are often otherwise unavailable. This method will provide a view from the user of the service and often gives an insight into both emotional and physical experiences, providing both qualitative and quantitative data; it can be used as part of the Step 1 process mapping exercise as well as during the testing and pilot stage.

This simple method requires the provision of a dated document that the patient holds throughout an agreed period of time, usually a time reflecting the period of the event subject to the change. A patient attending for a tonsillectomy, for example, would be invited to join the study at the first outpatient appointment, prior to seeing the clinical staff. The study would be explained and the person's participation secured. The patient would be requested to complete each page in the diary as events occurred. The events recorded might include a wide range of activities, from parking the car, understanding how to get to their destination, how and when personal details were taken and even the attitudes of staff.

The diaries should then be collated and the comments categorised. It is important at this stage not to dismiss any comments. In using this exercise in work undertaken in the re-engineering change project at the Leicester Royal Infirmary NHS Trust, it was identified, during a simple ENT process review, that one patient had had his personal details taken 14 times by different members of staff.

Patient interviews

To undertake interviews, it is essential to predetermine the structure and content of the interview framework. Interviews should always be semi-structured as patients will always want to 'tell it as it is', resulting in unique data. The questions should be agreed with the team, and an interview may take place both prior to and on completion of the patient's experience. The most useful way to record interviews of this nature is to use a tape recorder, having first secured the patient's agreement. This leaves the interviewer to listen to the patient and to document other activities such as body language or actions that will not be picked up on the tape recorder. The tape can then later be transcribed and the transcript collated with any notes taken.

Quantitative data collection

You may wish to derive some statistical evidence to support the change process, and such data can be obtained from many sources. The timing of events can usually be extracted from the medical and nursing case notes, for example, the date on which the referral was received, the date the first appointment was sent, the date of the appointment, the dates of admission and discharge, and the date the discharge letter was dispatched. This method can also be employed to identify the use of analgesia or other drugs, identifying the quantity and timing of administration.

It is important at this stage also to undertake a cost analysis; therefore it will be essential to employ the services of the organisation's financial advisors. Cost analysis may include staff time and equipment costs.

Qualitative analysis

A substantial number of data will be obtained from the patient diaries, but it is also essential to consider in this evaluation the feelings and experiences of the staff involved, which may be undertaken through a semi-structured interview process at the end of the pilot, again ensuring an agreed framework for the interview.

Step 4: Achieving the optimum

Having conducted the pilot and run an evaluation, the feasibility of implementation will be identifiable. Step 4 will highlight those areas which require further change or refinement and identify additional training and education needs. In more extreme circumstances, it is possible to identify physical and environmental changes.

1. Review and analyse the evaluation data collected via interviews and patient diaries.
2. Review and analyse the financial implications.
3. Remove any identifiable unnecessary components.

4. Determine the changes required that will make the process more effective and efficient
5. Achieve consensus on the part of all team members
6. Go to the implementation stage.

It must be recognised at this stage that it may be necessary to return to Step 2 of the process.

Step 5: Implementation

The success of this model requires an essential commitment to its implementation. Mechanisms are therefore required to support the implementation, with a clear identification of accountability, roles, skills, training, equipment and information requirements. It is essential to acknowledge that the success of sustainable change is dependent on teamwork, communication, cooperation and collaboration. The change process must be subjected to regular review over time to ensure that it continues to meet the needs of both the patient and the service. Finally, the most essential ingredient of all at this stage is to celebrate success. *Success is sweet and is the fuel of continued change and lifelong learning.*

Key Point Summary

- Establish a team
- Share values and goals
- Celebrate your success
- Constant refinement and evaluation are essential

2

Clinical Governance: a Framework and Models for Practice

Irene Scott

The term 'governance' has featured highly in recent years on the NHS agenda and has aimed to ensure excellence in the corporate governance and the financial governance of health institutions. In essence, the focus has been on the organisational management and financial probity of healthcare, resulting in control being focused on the managers of the systems. Today's approach to clinical governance has presented a new challenge to healthcare in embracing the very clinical professionals who are at the heart of healthcare delivery, in achieving excellence and in ensuring the very raison d'être of the NHS – equity of access, and equity of expected and anticipated outcome. This chapter discusses the development of clinical governance, its role in today's health system and its challenges to the professions and the institutions. In an aim to provide readers with an opportunity to explore their own position within clinical governance, I will discuss some commonly raised questions: What is clinical governance? How will we recognise it? How will we monitor and measure it? What is my role in clinical governance? What is clear at this point is that clinical governance is not necessarily tangible; it is a concept and a way of life, a way of life that requires a considerable change in the culture of healthcare and healthcarers, as described in Chapter 1.

What is governance?

The term 'governance' means the direction and control of the actions, affairs, policies and functions of an organisation, exercising restraint over, regulating, directing, determining or deciding something (*Collins Concise English Dictionary*, 1982). Therefore, if we preface this term with 'clinical', we can determine that clinical activity, that is, diagnosis, treatment and the delivery of care, will form the basis for all future actions and developments and will underpin the future of NHS.

Considering that the focus in healthcare in recent years has been on the financial agenda and managerial framework, we are presented with a challenge that demands a radical change in thinking, which will in essence require a fundamental change in culture. The drive from today's government is to build an NHS that is 'modern and dependable', 'fit for the twenty first century', a service that is based on need rather than on the ability to pay, who the GP is or where the individual may live (DoH, 1998b). This premise was set against the desire to 'abolish the internal market' (DoH, 1998b, p. 5, para 1.4), a system that has been the focus of healthcare institutions for the past nine years in its drive for cost-effectiveness and efficiency.

Using the 'retrospectorscope' we can plot the lifeline of governance to enable us to determine what has led us to today's model. It is interesting, however, to recognise that, since the inception of the NHS in 1948, much of the governance has been greatly influenced by the medical profession, in so far as the medical profession was able to create an environment conducive to its own need at a time when Aneurin Bevan was working to produce a national system (see Chapter 1). This influence has remained throughout the development of the NHS, the Conservative government reforms of the 1980s reporting that the government 'underestimated the power of doctors to resist challenges to their traditional way of doing things' (Harrison et al., 1992, p. 2).

It can be seen that, throughout the 1970s and 80s and into the 1990s, the focus of health system redesign was on models of management. The National Health Service Act of 1974 saw the introduction of Regional Hospital Boards and Hospital Management Committees, the Royal Commission of 1979 subsequently seeing a reduction in the number of management tiers. Then,

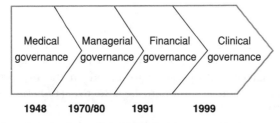

Figure 2.1 The evolution of governance (adapted from Scott, 1999)

in 1983, the Griffiths Report provided a focus for a greater cost-effectiveness and introduced the 'general management' function. The major concern at this time was to keep within budget (Ham, 1992), the argument being that hospital doctors should accept a greater responsibility for keeping costs in line with the budget. Under the same government, this then led quite naturally to the reforms of 1991 with the publication of the White Paper *Working for Patients* (DoH, 1998a), which introduced the Trust management system with self-managed units and purchasing and providing. The agenda was thereby clearly to become focused on financial efficiency, which has been the most recent driver of healthcare. The evolution of governance (Figure 2.1) has now quite rightly drawn the service to a position in which the future NHS can put the patient at the heart of development, and healthcare providers will for the first time hold a statutory duty for quality improvement.

Clinical governance – everyone's agenda

Clinical governance was first discussed in *A First Class Service – Quality in the New NHS* (DoH, 1998a, p. 9). It is described as:

> the process by which each part of the NHS quality assures its clinical decisions. Backed by a new statutory duty of quality it will introduce a system of continuous improvement into the operation of the whole NHS. Clinical governance, for example, will provide a means for hospitals to identify and address weaknesses in post operative care.

The drive behind this statement was 'to place quality at the heart of healthcare' (DoH, 1998a, p. 2). This clearly aims to ensure qualitative working rather than simply quantitative working using the practice of 'ticking boxes'. The aim is to provide a service that will continually improve the overall standard of clinical care, reduce the variations in outcomes of access to service, as well as ensure that clinical decisions are based on the most up-to-date evidence of what is known to be effective (*Clinical Governance*, DoH, 1998).

Three main elements have been determined to underpin this development, sitting principally at two levels, the national and the local:

1. The setting of clear national quality standards through National Service Frameworks (NSFs) and the NICE.

2. Local clinical governance frameworks for ensuring the local delivery of high-quality clinical services through Health Improvement Programmes (HIMPs), supported by a process of appropriately designed education and therefore 'lifelong' learning.

3. Effective systems for monitoring the delivery of quality standards through local audit and a new statutory body that is being formed at the time of writing – the Commission for Health Improvement (see Figure 2.2).

National level

National Service Frameworks

To ensure and facilitate the development of equitable, high-quality services across the country, NSFs are being developed, starting in high-priority areas. It could be argued that the first of these frameworks, although not referred to as such at the time, was encapsulated in the Calman Hine Report on cancer services (DoH, 1995). The report made recommendations to ensure a parity of services for all cancer patients regardless of where they might reside, and to ensure the maximum possible cure rate and best quality of life (DoH, 1995). It recognised the need to ensure that clinical expertise underpinned practice at all levels in both the primary and secondary care sectors. This report set the scene for future NSFs such as the *National Service Framework*

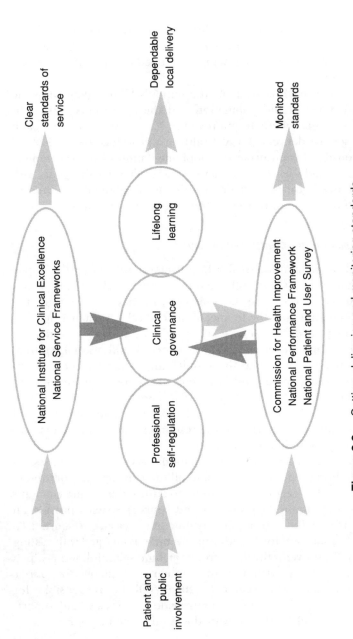

Figure 2.2 Setting, delivering and monitoring standards (DoH, 1998a, p. 8)

for Mental Health (DoH, 1999b) and the *National Service Framework for Coronary Heart Disease* (DoH, 2000a), while frameworks are at the time of writing being developed for care of the elderly and diabetes.

This approach is arguably the nation's HIMP, identifying the health need of the population and the approach required by healthcare providers to improve the state of the nation's health and service delivery. Local healthcare providers are to be held responsible for ensuring the implementation of the recommendations made in these frameworks and aligning the goals with local need and the values of the local population, thereby creating a change process within the local environment.

Commission for Health Improvement

The Commission for Health Improvement will review the implementation of NSFs at both a national and a local level in relation to clinical governance. Its aims are to review and monitor the implementation of the totality of the clinical governance agenda, and to provide a resource to support healthcare providers in the development of clinical governance. It will also target areas of difficulty, undertake the monitoring of local clinical governance arrangements and intervene in service development and implementation at the request of the Secretary of State (DoH, 1998a, p. 51). In the practice of today's administration, it will make public its reports and the responses and recommendations made by those bodies examined.

To ensure a comprehensive national system, it will be essential to bring together the work of all the existing statutory monitoring bodies (Figure 2.3), aiming to ensure that all the elements of an organisation's processes and support systems provide an opportunity for assuring quality outcome measures (Figure 2.4). The Commission for Health Improvement is charged with visiting every Trust over a three- or four-year time span, following which reports will be written with summaries available for public consumption. The regional offices will be responsible for following up the action plans provided to Trusts, and reports and plans will be shared with the Audit Commission.

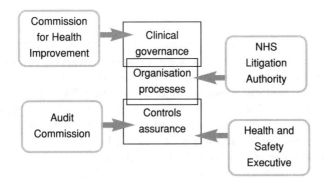

Figure 2.3   National bodies informing and
monitoring organisational risk

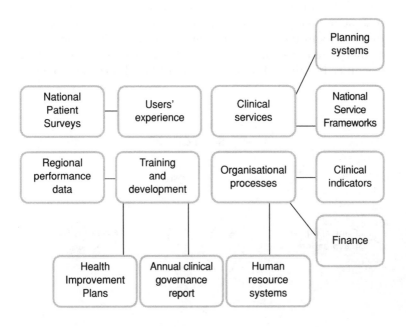

Figure 2.4   Routine information that will be required
to inform performance monitoring

The National Institute for Clinical Excellence

While it is true to say that much medical treatment has been subjected to research, producing evidence for practice, it is arguable that there remains a vast variation in treatment, and even where the evidence exists, little is in use. The framework for clinical effectiveness recommended by the NHS Executive (Figure 2.5) starts and ends with identifying good practice, integrating evidence with clinical audit, and research. Yet it remains a fact that, notwithstanding over £500 million having been invested in clinical audit activity over the past eight years, most Trusts would have difficulty in identifying the value of this investment.

It is arguable that this funding was a prime inducement to the medical profession at the time of implementing the White Paper *Working for Patients* (DoH, 1990) in 1991. It is also true to say that it is difficult to locate in the literature any indication of the evidence-based practice used by the nursing profession that is measurable in its implementation. Furthermore, while medical treatment has enjoyed the fruits of research, not only in changing treatment and the process of diagnosis, but also in its serving to further raise the status of the profession, it could be argued that few other health professions or areas of healthcare have enjoyed

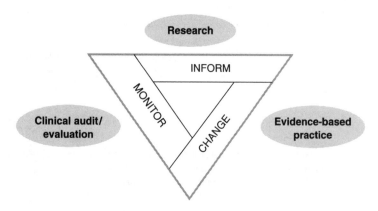

Figure 2.5   The NHS recommended framework for clinical effectiveness, requiring an integrated approach
(adapted from NHS Executive, 1996a)

the same attention. There is little evidence to support the delivery of care by any professional group, or indeed the organisation of care, perhaps because much of this work could be conceded to be subjective (the very nature of qualitative research) and therefore not an attractive financial investment for funding bodies. After all, although there is money to be made in the drug market, there is none to be made, or little, in changes in care practices or organisational structuring.

The NICE has been established to set standards by developing clinical guidelines based on evidence of clinical and cost-effectiveness, to agree associated clinical audit methodologies and to inform on good practice. Its intention is to play a major role in producing guidelines for the use of significant and new and existing interventions, such as the introduction of new drugs and treatments. It is perhaps arguable that this body will in the future extend its remit, working closely with the Commission for Health Improvement, to identify and disseminate evidence-based organisation of care and organisational management.

Local level

Healthcare providers are responsible for implementing the recommendations of the NSFs as well as for developing local services that reflect the needs of the local population through HIMPs. HIMPs are established by the involvement and participation of all care sectors, including primary care, secondary care and social care, and where possible local education systems and in some cases local industry. Individual HIMPs employ the clinical expertise of professional groups and develop plans to deliver a service that aims ultimately to improve the health of the local population, in terms of, for example, diabetes, coronary heart disease, stroke and child health. The need will be determined by the health of the population, which will obviously be influenced by demography. It has been clearly demonstrated that the demographic picture varies widely: where there is a large group of one ethnic origin, for example, the healthcare need will differ. Leicester houses a large Asian population (28 per cent in the inner city compared with 11 per cent county-wide), with a high incidence of diabetes. In other areas with a high middle-class

Caucasian population, there may be a high incidence of coronary heart disease. The local HIMPs will need to identify targets and significant resource needs and be underpinned by professional education.

It is clear then that many agencies and many professionals will be required to build and deliver the agreed targets. The nursing and care agenda will inevitably be greatly implicated in this by identifying both role and opportunity and must therefore position itself both to influence and to respond to changes in practice. It is not enough simply to pay lip service to the breaking down of professional barriers. The profession must identify how it is best placed to deliver the care agenda and in doing so recognise the need to ensure that a high level of education is available to underpin practice. Clinical activity must not be guarded jealously by the professions. Care must be delivered at the most appropriate time by the most appropriate person, be that a registered practitioner, a healthcare support worker or a social care worker.

This new focus on quality in the NHS will clearly demand participation and partnership working from all groups who contribute to the health and social care agenda and to the creation of 'an environment in which excellence will flourish' (DoH, 1998a). To produce this environment, we need to recognise and understand just what clinical governance is and what this means to the professionals working under it. It will obviously affect all the professions and will become the very basis of their working lives. Backed by the new statutory duty, its aim is to introduce a system of continuous quality improvement, and it will therefore be implicitly underpinned by a process of lifelong learning in order to ensure that NHS staff have 'the tools and the knowledge to offer the most modern, effective and high quality care to patients' (DoH, 1998a).

Establishing an effective clinical governance framework that is meaningful to both staff and patients has stretched professional imaginations, quite simply because they have been grappling with a concept rather than a prescriptive approach, thereby leaving the interpretation of the requirements of a clinical governance framework to the individual healthcare organisation. Whatever the framework, it is arguable that, in order to avoid a quantitative approach to ensuring quality, it is not enough simply to set up

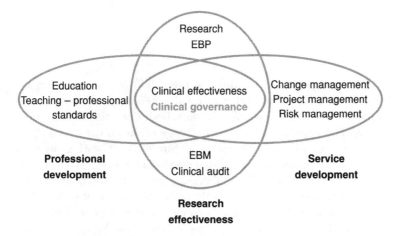

Figure 2.6 inner content:

Research
EBP

Education
Teaching – professional
standards

Clinical effectiveness
Clinical governance

Change management
Project management
Risk management

**Professional
development**

EBM
Clinical audit

**Service
development**

**Research
effectiveness**

Existing elements must inform and influence each other

EBM = evidence-based management; EBP = evidence-based practice

Figure 2.6   Key components of a clinical
governance model (adapted from Scott, 1999)

new committees. The success of a clinical governance framework
depends upon the ability of existing elements to inform and influence each other (Scott, 1999), and many of these elements already
exist in every organisation, albeit to varying degrees (Figure 2.6).

The Leicester Royal Infirmary NHS Trust took the above
approach to developing a clinical governance framework in an
aim to enlist all its staff members, recognising that each member,
whether a clinical professional, a secretary or a porter, plays a
key role in the delivery of quality care. The approach taken was
iterative in nature, thereby creating a learning environment and
recognising failure as part of its development. The key components were recognised as being:

- Research
- Education and training
- Clinical and organisational audit
- Change management skills
- Evidence-based clinical practice

- Evidence-based managerial practice
- Risk management
- Project management skills.

The complementary nature of these skills enabled the organisation to determine and provide the necessary information to enable it to measure its effectiveness, both operationally and clinically. The approach created a marriage of the strategic and operational agenda, offering an opportunity to all staff groups to influence professional and service development need. What is clear in this model is that staff members cannot react without an appropriate level of information. It is therefore essential that good information is available for all the elements. It is arguable that the informed will enhance and change practice based on information demonstrating variables, such as benchmarking against similar processes of care and outcomes of care. It is, after all, human nature to aspire to be at least equal to one's counterparts.

It must be recognised, however, that major change, such as that demanded by the clinical governance model, will not occur by simply introducing the concept to staff and expecting the results to be realised. The very nature of the national healthcare system has enabled tradition and ritual to perpetuate, one generation passing down its lessons to the next and thus creating a culture of 'the way we do things around here'. The organisation and the individuals in it must learn to think and act differently, which can only be facilitated by ownership of change at the highest level.

Trust boards and senior healthcare leaders such as chief executives and directors must first recognise the need to change and the need to empower staff, creating a learning environment that generates accountability and continuous learning. The organisation must be given the skills to recognise and execute its capability. To this end, the Leicester Royal Infirmary established a Centre for Best Practice, a learning centre in which skills could be disseminated to clinical teams. These skills primarily focused on change management skills, which underpinned the redesign of working practices, empowering staff to influence the delivery of care in their local environment. In essence, the very culture of the Trust was moved from that of tradition and function to that of innovation and patient process.

Challenges and clinical governance

It is clear that the new agenda is complex, not least in its demands to develop a new way of thinking and therefore a new culture. A paradigm shift is required to move the control of past management structures closer to the delivery of care, and, as argued by Neubauer (1997), people must now learn to manage and take responsibility for their own actions and their own careers, rather than depending on a paternalistic organisation to do this for them. However, to engage everyone in this agenda and ensure a co-commitment in service development and delivery, excellence in leadership throughout the continuum of care must be enabled.

Recognising that leadership does not equal hierarchy, Neubauer (1997) argues that leadership in developing organisations is not a control system, but an influence. Developing organisations are rarely tidy structures and are more likely to appear messy as they are based around visionary development rather than problem-solving. It is difficult to draw the structure of an organisation that is empowering as there are no or few lines of direct accountability, and the hierarchy is hardly tangible.

My first experience of this was in attempting to draw the organisational structure of the Leicester Royal Infirmary, which resembled a very complex wiring diagram. The self-managed process teams were identifiable as organisations in their own right, but to function effectively they had to be interdependent with many departments that had co-opted team membership. Multiply this framework several times and this gives you a single directorate structure; multiply this again several times and you have the organisation structure. The very essence of this approach ensures accountability at all levels and demands the involvement of all staff in determining the goals of the organisation and therefore the strategic direction. A failure on the part of leadership to recognise this involvement will generate an organisation that pulls in different directions and creates chaos in achieving equity of care for its patient population.

There is a sea of text available talking about leadership and management, much of which provides lists of characteristics that appear to be common to whatever one is leading. Bennis (1993), in his work studying the great leaders, likened leaders of the arts to leaders of corporations, indicating a belief that leadership traits are the same regardless of profession. It is clear, however, that in leadership today, in order to ensure leadership at all levels, skills must be adjusted proportionally to the situation, the competencies and skills being matched to the life cycle of the business and the position of the strategy. While Smith Blancett and Flarey (1995) argue that leaders emerge, we cannot antici- pate that there is an inbuilt leader in every team. Today's agenda demands leadership, so the designated leader must possess skills in accordance with the desires and aims of the team in order to enable and facilitate a consensus of goal alignment. This argu- ment is supported by Hammer and Champy (1993, p. 105), who argue that in a change environment 'a caretaker of the status quo will never be able to muster the passion and enthusiasm the effort requires'. The leader in a change environment is required to motivate and influence the team he or she works within.

The common themes emanating from the literature suggest that leaders make people want to follow them (Bennis, 1985; Kets de Vries, 1993). Authors of leadership comment that leaders should have, among other skills, vision, good communication skills and energy (Bennis, 1985; Hammer and Champy, 1993; Kets de Vries, 1993); however, to influence change and to empower teams, personal characteristics must come into play. Kets de Vries (1993) describes what I believe are three of the most valuable human and personal attributes of a leader – humility, humanity and humour – arguing that such qualities as these can prevent excessive organisational neurosis and contribute to organisational stability. It is true to say that any leaders who are able to recog- nise their own failings and support others in theirs will create an environment of trust and a desire to be involved. Yet perhaps one of this most fundamental of all attributes is the ability to find humour in what we do, to have fun and to enjoy not only our work, but also each other's contributions and style. While many of those perceived to be leaders in today's NHS are artic- ulate and visionary, and work long hours, there is evidence to suggest that they have greater difficulty in achieving corporate success than those who possess the ability to build teams and empower team members (Kets de Vries, 1993).

The term 'empowerment' is frequently found in the literature when discussing leadership, being described as the process of enabling an individual or a team to act as it believes most approp-

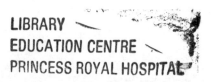

riate in meeting its goals and to making its own decisions (Bennis, 1985; Kets de Vries, 1993). In terms of healthcare, however, the team comprises a main body of what we may determine to be powerful healthcare professionals. The power may be that of the dominant doctor or the control exerted by a manager. The largest participating group in a healthcare team is, however, likely to be nurses, with a smaller number of doctors and other occupational groups. Therefore, to enable team empowerment, all players must subscribe to the same goals, yet this may be tempered by the power of professional groups and a conflict between values of personal autonomy and team goals.

Given the change required to meet the goals of clinical governance, it is not enough to be a leader with vision, good communication skills and energy. Much of the change agenda will only be achieved through an iterative approach, planning, implementing and evaluating a change process. What is clear is that change is not always successful and depends upon many factors. Today's leaders are therefore required to have, above all, optimism. An optimistic approach to change enables the leader to view failure as lessons to be learned and remain charged with enthusiasm to achieve the team vision and create continuous improvement.

Risk management and clinical governance

My various roles in healthcare in recent years have brought me into contact with many healthcare organisations and agencies, and it is interesting to note that many individuals see clinical governance simply as a risk management framework, thereby creating fear in clinical practice. This has generated a concept of 'am I doing the right thing right?' There is a recognition that the accountability of practitioners is being called into question: it is no longer satisfactory to determine a reason for action as 'we have always done it this way'. It is clear that risk management is fundamental to the success of the clinical governance agenda, yet it cannot stand alone. There is probably a risk in everything we do, from recruiting staff to delivering care. Organisational risk management structures must be robust and form a distinct part of any clinical governance framework, involving all staff and being seen to be informing both the audit and the research agenda.

A good and simple example of risk management is the monitoring of complaints. An organisation that monitors complaints well can identify common concerns and common areas of failure. This information can in turn be used to generate focused audit activities, enabling a breadth and depth of understanding of the nature and extent of the failure. The results of the audit may determine a research process that will in turn identify standards. Agreed standards may then be implemented and an evaluation/audit process set up after an agreed period. The nature of this process enables both organisational and individual learning.

The reality of healthcare is that it is delivered by people of varying expertise with varying expectations. It is therefore no surprise that we commonly deal with poor performance. Poorly performing healthcare professionals are a risk not only to patients, but also to the organisations for which they work. While these individuals are relatively few in number, their existence poses a problem that must be addressed in order to ensure excellence in clinical care and the confidence on the part of the public.

The sole purpose of clinical governance is clearly not to sort out poorly performing professionals, yet it does create a drive to ensure that poor practice is rectified. In recognition of the importance of ensuring a high standard of practice and the identification of poor practice, the professional bodies are moving to a regulation of the professions that enables poor performance to be measured against agreed competencies and standards of practice rather than the proponents simply being protected by their fellow professionals. The test for the service will be, as Scally and Donaldson (1998) describe, in dealing with cases in a sympathetic manner, which, while correctly putting the protection of patients first, will also deal fairly with experienced and highly trained professionals. It must be recognised, however, that those who knowingly ignore or pass on a poorly performing individual from one organisation to another by the delivery of reasonable or good references are as culpable of bad practice as those whom they are referencing.

Research underpinning effectiveness

Research in the creation of evidence is core to the delivery of effective practice. If nurses and related professions are to have a major impact on the clinical governance agenda, they must, like their medical counterparts, invest both time and energy in undertaking research and transferring its findings into practice. It is clear that the nursing profession recognises the value of both carrying out and implementing research, yet it has to rise to the challenge to realise its full potential. It must gain a confidence in not only disseminating research findings and implementing evidence-based practice, but also recognising its ability to undertake research. The majority of nurses practising today were trained in a traditional system, and while those nurses trained and educated through the Project 2000 diploma system have been taught the principles of analysis and evaluation, the former group have not been given these skills. It is thus essential that nurses develop such proficiency to enable the assessment of studies that may be judged and applied to the relevance of local need (Boden and Kelly, 1999).

Boden and Kelly recognise how the small-scale nature of clinical nursing research has placed it in a low position in the hierarchy of healthcare studies, yet nursing research has a potentially untapped source: its very nature of clinical activity, which many nurses use on a daily basis to test out the effectiveness of various practices in a variety of situations. They are in essence performing action research. This research approach, known as 'praxis', is action informed by practical theory and is defined by Wheeler and Chinn (1984, p. 2) as 'thoughtful reflection and action that occur in synchrony, in the direction of the transforming world'. Rolfe (1996) identifies the term 'praxis' as having its origins in Greece, where it was used by Aristotle to describe a doing action and describes how Marx adopted the term to denote the unity of theory and practice.

In light of this explanation, imagine the richness of data that could become available if nursing documented and shared its research findings. Boden and Kelly (1999) recognise and support the action of taking the results of effectiveness measures as a starting point, assessing the available evidence base and then initiating research that has a direct relevance to local health need, the outcome of which would be a demonstrable change in the scope of nursing research. This approach may be seen to support and enhance the value of research as praxis, recognising the essence of nursing practice as the content of nursing research. Nursing now has to change its mindset with relation to not only how research is performed and disseminated, but also how it positions itself to gain access to the wide availability of research funding. While this shift may take time, it is essential to capitalise on the clinical governance agenda and aim to embed evidence into clinical practice, ensuring equity in the continuing debate on this governance model, which ensures that evidence informs policy appropriately.

Nursing must now recognise that, to fulfil its full potential in the clinical governance agenda, it needs to gain a stronger position in the research world. Clinical governance is the opportunity the profession has been waiting for; it gives licence to aim high and change and strengthen its current status. While much nursing research has operated outside the mainstream of healthcare, we must now learn to exploit this new opportunity and bring research into daily practice. Boden and Kelly (1999, p. 186) however, issue a cautionary note in that 'there is little reason to expect that nursing research will strengthen its position, either in terms of status or increased investment, without it first providing the evidence that nursing research can yield benefit to the NHS'.

Closing the loop – using pathways as a means of achieving clinical governance

A question we must ask ourselves with regard to progressing and participating in the development of clinical governance is surely 'how will we know when we have it?' This question generates the further, perhaps more profound, question of 'will we ever truly achieve clinical governance and equity of access for all?' (DoH, 1998a). These questions are true imponderables given that, as a national institution, we will always have power bases in one place or another, and hierarchy will remain a fact of life. Life itself has a hierarchy, and many individuals are comfortable living within a hierarchy, as it creates a comfortable environment in which accountability is limited to those in power. Having articulated this, one would anticipate that the optimist will always see an opportunity to reach for something new, and create continuous learning and therefore continuous quality improvement.

In recent years many approaches have been taken in an attempt to achieve continuous quality improvement: more recently, we have been made familiar with 'care pathways', processes of care and patient journeys. It could be argued that they are one and the same thing in that they all aim to provide parity and equity of care that is efficient and cost-effective. However, the clinical governance model dictates that it is no longer adequate to have an agreed pathway of care if it is not underpinned by evidence, research, appropriate skills and competencies, and aims for agreed outcomes. Neither is it adequate to plan a patient's care singularly for the institution.

The literature describes many models of pathways of care. American models of such pathways have been underpinned by the desire to improve efficiency as a first priority, while the UK approach has been to ensure agreed outcomes of care with equity of access to services for the population for whom it is providing. It is clearly essential to determine what a pathway of care is and, in doing so, recognise its congruence with clinical governance.

While Wilson (1997) describes pathways of care as 'producing the best prescribed outcomes within resources and activities available for an appropriate episode of care', we may choose to question what constitutes an episode of care. Where does it begin, and where does it end? If we are to discuss total patient care and truly achieve excellence, it must be recognised that care does not begin and end at the institutional walls. The pathway is generally described as beginning when the patient enters the secondary care system and ending in his or her return to primary care.

However, if we are to ensure excellence and equity of care and outcomes, it is surely essential to encompass all care sectors (thereby avoiding an unnecessary delay in transfer), variables in treatment and parity of outcome. A care pathway is not simply about ensuring that clinical records and documentation are available for and used by a multi-disciplinary team. Johnson (1995) describes the development of integrated care pathways as a quality improvement tool that is a multi-disciplinary case management tool and clinical audit tool. This tool identifies nursing and medical activities that must occur in a consecutive and synchronised fashion in order to achieve the desired outcomes throughout an appropriate episode of care. All authors of pathways espouse the essential ingredient as being the multi-disciplinary team, and that surely cannot be argued with.

Box 2.1

**Opportunities to address all aspects
of clinical governance**

A care pathway is an excellent tool for enabling the clinical governance agenda, recognising:

- multi-professional care delivery
- the implementation of evidence
- the provision of an audit trail
- the identification and reduction of the opportunity for risk
- the identification of an opportunity for new research

The development of a care pathway is a true opportunity to address all aspects of the clinical governance agenda (Box 2.1).

In developing care pathways, everyone who is likely to participate in care, however small their contribution may be, must be involved in its design. In essence the pathway must be owned by those who are to deliver it in order to ensure the highest quality. However, it is simply not enough to obtain support at all levels: the process design must recognise many opportunities (Box 2.2), not least the opportunity to identify the need to introduce

---

Box 2.2

**Pathways as an opportunity to identify
developments in practice and education**

Care pathways create an opportunity to:

- identify good practice
- remove bad practice
- design a bespoke service
- identify and implement evidence-based practice
- identify education and training needs
- appreciate the skills and contributions of all the professions and care sectors involved

---

evidence-based practice, where evidence exists, and recognise the relevant areas for future research activity. It must serve to sift out all elements of risk and identify the appropriate skills and competencies of those who are to deliver the component parts.

Here, there is also an opportunity to identify the person or persons best placed to deliver that care, who may not always be the professionals traditionally trained for the practice. This creates both a personal and a professional development opportunity for individuals, enabling a broadening of the scope of individual practice. Changes in skill and competency clearly require appropriate education and training. It is therefore essential to include educational institutions in the development of pathways. The implementation of pathways requires great skill in change management, and if these skills are not employed participants may simply carry on in the same way as they have in the past.

The effect of sustaining change must not go unrecognised as a key success factor of care pathways. Throughout the development of a care pathway, it is essential to consider how the loop may be closed (Figure 2.7). Audit and evaluation mechanisms must be agreed and implemented, as it is only by using audit and evaluation methods that one can determine the success of the activities involved and identify the need for refinement and change.

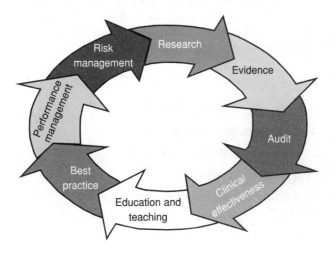

Figure 2.7 The core elements of clinical governance creating the basis for good care pathways

Summary

Clinical governance can arguably be seen as the most timely development in healthcare, creating as the focus of the delivery of care the patient rather than those delivering the service. It is a framework that creates many challenges and stretches the imagination. It is a time and an opportunity to think 'new', to challenge the norm and to demonstrate effectiveness in both clinical care and organisational design. The elements of clinical governance exist in every organisation. It is not new and it is not 'rocket science'; it is a means of ensuring that each participating element interfaces with and informs the next. It is no longer satisfactory for developments to exist in a vacuum or indeed for individuals to act in a vacuum.

The success of clinical governance depends on all the participants recognising and taking responsibility for their own contribution and being accountable for their actions. The identification and development of evidence-based practice must not be committed to the shelves of academia but shared and implemented across the service. Individuals must recognise their role in ensuring that practice is based on evidence and, where the evidence does not exist, taking responsibility for finding it. The agenda is a shared one and is reliant upon good teamwork in which teams share goals and values, and excellent leadership in an environment that generates learning and recognises opportunity and challenge as a key to improvement.

Key Point Summary

▓ Clinical governance is not rocket science

▓ Clinical governance aims to ensure excellence

▓ It embraces clinical care

▓ It will ensure access and equity of access

3

Research and Evidence-based Practice

Dawn Freshwater and Rebecca Broughton

The development of nursing theory and the acknowledgement of the differing sources of knowledge has brought to a head the argument that nursing theory and nursing practice must be founded on a scientific basis (Akinsanya, 1985; Osbourne, 1991; Salvage, 1998). The phrase 'evidence based' is increasingly entering the discourse on effectiveness in nursing (Bonnell, 1999; Closs and Cheater, 1999) and has captured the attention of both managers and researchers alike, the former because of its seeming potential to rationalise costs in healthcare provision, the latter because of its association with problems related to the lack of adoption of research findings in nursing. Evidence-based practice is, however, not just about ensuring that practice is substantiated by research; it is also concerned with accountable practice and as such requires that practitioners make their private knowledge public. This chapter considers the challenges posed to nursing practice of not only how to get research into practice, thereby ensuring that nursing care is founded upon the best available evidence, but also achieving this from a stance of professional accountability and responsibility.

One of the main difficulties of writing a chapter such as this is that of demonstrating the integration of research literature (and therein role modelling the inextricable connection of theory, practice and research) while at the same time making the text accessible and relevant to readers. It is true that many clinical nurses feel that academic research is of little relevance to them, and even if the research is answering a practice-based question,

the findings still have to be communicated in an understandable way. Thus, as the authors of this chapter, we find ourselves
experiencing the struggle that we are now to write about. So
while the chapter incorporates research evidence, it is written
from a subjective standpoint, and we must leave it to readers to
validate and interpret the text in their own way. In the true
sense of practice-based research, this is the only way to validate
the findings.

That nursing ought be founded on a scientific basis is not a
new proposition: Chater in 1975, for example, not only maintained
that nursing should be underpinned by scientific principles, but
also added that patient care should be founded on defensible,
research-based findings. Dramatic changes in healthcare and the
rapid growth of care pathways and integrated care delivery systems
have focused practitioners' attention on enhancing patient
outcomes through providing effective nursing practice. It has been
argued that *not* to base nursing practice on research is unethical
(Styles, 1982), but how does one overcome the barriers to the
application, dissemination and uptake of research findings that
continue to plague the world of nursing? For while it is acknowledged that nursing practice should be based on the best available evidence, and it is fair to say that there are now more
opportunities for developing and increasing nursing research than
ever before, nursing care and treatment remains largely unaffected
by research findings (Walshe et al., 1995; Coombs, 1999).

Applying research findings in nursing practice is perhaps one
of the biggest challenges facing nursing research and the development of the profession (Le May et al., 1998; Tierney, 1998).
This is not to say that there is a general disinterest in research
approaches and methods on the part of nurses. Indeed, nursing
research is becoming more established (witness the plethora of
research papers in the nursing literature), and there is little
doubt that there is an increased interest in the variety of research
approaches and their theoretical perspectives.

While being actively engaged in the debate concerning the epis-
temological and the methodological credibility of research
approaches to nursing is commendable, it would seem that the
debate itself could be limiting as the task of implementation
becomes subsumed in a discussion that concentrates on polar-
ising methodological models. Arguably, what is contestable is the

value of nursing research that does not affect treatment and care. In order to facilitate the use of research findings and to ensure that nursing practice is founded on the best available evidence, nursing practice has been assigned the task of implementing evidence-based practice (DoH, 1989a). Evidence-based practice demands that nurses maintain a closer compatibility between their nursing beliefs and their nursing care. How can nursing best respond to these challenges and changes? What is required to enable nursing, midwifery and health visiting to seek out the best evidence, personalise it and apply it to the local situation?

By way of addressing these and other related questions, we will first outline our understanding of the terms 'research' and 'evidence-based practice'. Barriers to improving clinical effectiveness through research will be examined alongside some of the contemporary developments, such as clinical governance and clinical supervision, in nursing and healthcare. Issues such as the theory–practice gap and practitioner-generated theory will be contextualised within a research framework, and recommendations will be made for practitioners wishing to take up the challenge posed. Clinical examples will be used to help to illustrate the practical application of the somewhat abstract concept of evidence-based practice. In conclusion, it will be argued that research grounded in practice has far better potential for improving the effectiveness and the knowledge base of nursing practice than research which is abstract from practice (Le May et al., 1998; Rolfe, 1998). Returning to the questions we have posed, it will be posited that local ownership is key to the successful implementation of research and therein evidence-based practice.

Research – the quest

Research has been described in many different ways, and there are numerous definitions to be found in the literature. Burns and Grove (1987, p. 4) define research as 'diligent, systematic inquiry or investigation to validate old knowledge and generate new knowledge'.

The Department of Health (1993, p. 6), for their contribution, state that 'Research is rigorous and systematic enquiry' that is 'designed to lead to generalisable contributions to knowledge'. Rolfe (1998), in his analysis of the many descriptions of research, suggests that the common theme that can be derived from the available definitions is that research is about generating knowledge. Knowledge can be generated in any number of ways, some methods attracting more credibility than others.

Miller and Crabtree (1999) identify five styles of research enquiry: experimental, survey, documentary–historical, field and philosophic. These styles fall along a continuum ranging from quantitative at one end, which favours control and prediction, to qualitative at the other end, which is idiographic and more interested in understanding and explaining. The choice of research style for a specific project depends upon the overarching aim of the research but will be heavily influenced by the preferred methodology of the researcher, the availability of resources, the time frame and other associated practicalities.

The main aim of clinical research is to identify best practice, with the purpose of adding to a general body of (generalisable) scientific knowledge, which can be shared with the larger scientific community as well as practitioners, managers and other professions allied to medicine. Thus clinical research has a tendency towards the quantitative end of the continuum. However, not all research (or practice) can be generalised (Closs and Cheater, 1996; Rolfe, 1998), which has had the effect of setting up a polemic between two seemingly opposing approaches. Whatever approach is taken, the researcher is an extremely important component of any research effort, the researcher's purposes, intentions and goals contributing significantly to the design, process and outcome of the research study.

In some of the more contemporary qualitative approaches to research design, there is a democratisation of the research endeavour. The researcher's status is not privileged over that of the participants, who may be referred to as co-researchers/investigators. This fits well with the recent trend towards consumer involvement in research (NHSE, 1998a), which emphasises 'active involvement of consumers in the research process, rather than the use of consumers as the "subjects" of research' (p. 4).

As already mentioned, qualitative and quantitative approaches to research have often been viewed as deriving from opposing philosophies of science, the debate surrounding the potential merits and shortcomings of quantitative and qualitative research being as much rehearsed in nursing as it is in all social sciences (Duffy, 1985; Webb, 1996). Qualitative methodology is often contrasted with quantitative research methodology in the nursing literature, and as such this chapter does not seek to repeat the differences between the two main approaches to enquiry; suffice it to say that each paradigm is associated with a specific methodology to gain knowledge (Mishler, 1979).

There is, instead, a more pressing issue of concern in the arena of nursing research, one that is more pertinent to the development of this book, that of enhancing the capability of staff to use research, both in practice and to change practice. As Tierney (1998) reports, the mere existence of research cannot change practice, the research has to be used. Many authors have expressed their concern about the apparent lack of impact that nursing research has made on practice (Bircumshaw, 1990; Le May et al., 1998) and the barriers that prevent its implementation.

Barriers to putting research into practice

A number of barriers to the effective adoption of research into practice have been identified, a trawl through the literature suggesting that there are four main factors influencing this process: access, attitude, institutional support and occupational culture (Hunt, 1987; Champion and Leach, 1989; Walczak et al., 1994). These four factors can be seen as leading to either organisational, cultural or methodological barriers (Le May et al., 1998; Coombs, 1999).

In a recent paper, Rafferty and Traynor (1999, p. 458) proposed that 'the NHS needs to create a research rich nursing culture if it is to influence the quality and outcomes of patient care'. This is fundamental to the development of professional and accountable nursing practice that is to be built upon a sound and appraised evidence base. Unfortunately, research is all too often seen to be someone else's role, some practitioners experiencing what one writer describes as a 'phobic reaction' to research (Mahood et al., 1995). This has not been helped by the DoH (1995) document outlining nursing's contribution to research and development, which states that research is a 'highly professional and specialised activity and not suited to every practitioner' (p. 2), which could be interpreted to mean that research is the domain of a specialist. While the document goes on to recommend that every practitioner needs to be involved in the utilisation of research results, it has the potential to perpetuate the belief that practitioner and researcher do not occupy the same world (Rolfe, 1998; Rafferty and Traynor, 1999).

As readers may be able to identify some of their own and indeed their colleagues' barriers to integrating research into everyday practice, some of the common themes that appear in the literature are outlined in the discussion that follows. Time constraints and heavy workloads are often given as organisational barriers to introducing new innovations in practice, but even when time is made available, nursing still has to contend with the deeply embedded negative attitudes and beliefs towards research (Hanson, 1994). Gadd et al. (1995) provide one example of such attitudes in their study revealing that reading research and visits to the library were often viewed as 'slacking off'. Several writers have discussed the importance of a positive attitude towards research. Lacey (1994), for example, found a positive correlation between attitudes to research and research utilisation; a positive attitude may help but the fact remains that few nurses actually make significant use of research findings in practice (Veeramah, 1995).

In order for nurses to develop a healthier attitude towards research, a strong infrastructure needs to be in place, one that provides significant experience not only of developing clinical guidelines, but also of fostering local adaptation to increase the ownership of relevant research findings. This needs to come before addressing the practical problems of time and workload constraints (something that is taken up in the current DoH (1999a) document *Making a Difference*).

The benefits, rewards and reinforcements that nurses receive for utilising research-based knowledge in practice need to be made explicit through increased institutional support. In other words, where you work must value research and its contribution to effective clinical care. Such a culture must flow from the board and cascade to all levels in the organisation.

Cultural barriers relate to the lack of preparation that practitioners receive for research in clinical practice. In the new health-care environment, practitioners must undertake the systematic review of research literature, the critical appraisal of research findings and the synthesis of empirical evidence with contextually relevant experience, that is, clinical experience and opinion-based processes. Practitioners often 'do' research as part of an academic course, which can provide some theoretical grounding in methods of searching and appraising research. Once back in practice, the knowledge and experience gained are not always followed through; in other words, results are rarely disseminated to colleagues, published locally and nationally, re-evaluated in the context of a developing clinical environment or presented at local research forums.

In addition, research that is undertaken as part of an educational course tends to focus on the course requirements rather than influencing local practice through researching local, regional and national initiatives, and such findings are not deemed relevant to practice so are not utilised (Yorkshire Regional Health Authority, 1991). The words 'vicious circle' come to mind. Greenwood (1984) concurs with this sentiment and argues that nurses do not find research findings relevant to their practice. She concludes that:

> Nursing is a practical activity, it is aimed at bringing about change in the physical, emotional and social status of persons – the problems that confront nurses are essentially practical problems concerning what to do. (p. 78)

A further barrier is the process of gaining ethical approval for research projects; a lengthy and sometimes medicalised process, it can feel obstructive to nurses interested in pursuing clinical research.

So while many nurses are aware of the importance of research findings, these are rarely applied. This is not surprising given the level of preparation that practitioners are afforded, for even published findings require the skills of interpretation and translation for their effective transference to the practitioner's own context and client group.

Methodological barriers centre around the quantitative/qualitative debate and the role of nursing research in the current NHS research and development (R&D) strategy (Tierney, 1998). Not all writers are caught up in this discussion: Salvage (1998) draws our attention to the political dimensions of the current

NHS R&D strategy, while Rafferty and Traynor (1999) discuss the lessons to be learnt from the research policy debate. It is clear that nurses need to be empowered to be able to join in this debate with confidence and see it as part of discharging their accountability and responsibility to their patients (Freshwater, 1999).

The current R&D strategy is informed by the hierarchy of evidence model (Long, 1998). The quality of evidence is assessed in terms of its level, knowledge gained through systematic review and randomised controlled trials being viewed as the most robust evidence. Many nurses do not feel comfortable with the idea of randomised controlled trials in nursing (Seers and Milne, 1997) as these do not always capture knowledge based in aesthetic experience and personal knowledge such as intuition. Herein lies a significant tension between nursing research and the current NHS R&D strategy's interpretation of evidence-based practice.

There are those who argue that knowledge is contingent, that research questions emerge after a period of familiarity within a specific setting and that, as such, practitioners are best placed to ask research questions (Fox, 1999). Hence research questions should be developed in such a way that the theoretical consequences will be of direct practical relevance, the appropriate methodology being employed to operationalise the research question.

A final point on methodological barriers relates to the lack of understanding of the differences between research and audit and their inherent processes. There continues to be a level of confusion among clinical nurses, and indeed some researchers and auditors, over the similarities and differences between audit and research (Closs and Cheater, 1996). This chapter does not seek to detail the differences, but it is worth noting that there is a distinct difference between the two, although both have links with quality and ensuring good practice. For an overview of the differences between audit and research, readers are directed to Closs and Cheater (1996).

Evidence-based practice

The literature surrounding evidence-based practice originates in medicine and implies a strong orientation towards randomised controlled trials, 'best evidence' being synonymous with empirical research or scientific evidence (Sackett et al., 1996; French, 1999). There are many definitions of evidence-based practice, evidence-based healthcare, evidence-based nursing and the forerunner of them all – evidence-based medicine, some of them more 'user friendly' than others. Sackett et al. (1996, p. 62) talk about the 'conscientious, explicit and judicious use of current best evidence'. Hicks (cited in Sackett et al.) includes 'due weight accorded to all valid relevant information' in his definition of evidence-based healthcare and 'using contemporaneous research findings' is part of Rosenberg and of Donald's (1995) definition of evidence-based medicine.

It is said that the purpose of evidence-based medicine is to 'base medical decisions on the best available evidence' (Sackett and Rosenberg, 1995, p. 64). Best *medical* practice has long been determined by the use of randomised controlled trials, and, as such, evidence-based *nursing* practice is a by-product of the modernist–rationalistic model, the dominant paradigm of the medical profession. The current paradigm shift that is taking place throughout the Western world in science means that the rationalistic, positivistic science is no longer the dominant worldview. Nursing is not a linear process and, while the nursing process has attempted (unsuccessfully we might argue) to order decision-making in nursing, it cannot order the world of the patient, which is non-linear, acausal and often chaotic (Marks-Maran, 1999). Nursing decisions are often made in random, intuitive ways based, it would seem, on personal opinion, professional expertise and an interpretation of the immediate context. Hence nursing must find an understanding of evidence-based practice that is congruent with its own philosophies and beliefs, and that fits with the emerging paradigm shift (Marks-Maran, 1999).

Since the introduction of evidence-based practice to the UK, another term has appeared – clinical effectiveness – and it is very often difficult to see whether these are separate activities or one and the same thing. Clinical effectiveness is defined by the NHS Executive (NHSE, 1996a, p. 3) as:

the extent to which specific clinical interventions, when deployed in the field for a particular patient or population, do what they are intended to do, that is, maintain and improve health and secure the greatest possible health gain from the available resources.

This definition has led some to think that clinical effectiveness is just another term for cost-effectiveness. The Royal College of Nursing (RCN) has adapted the NHSE's definition to formulate its own:

applying the best available knowledge for research, clinical expertise and patient preferences to achieve optimum processes and outcomes of care for patients. (RCN, 1998b)

The underlying aim in promoting clinical effectiveness is to ensure that, wherever possible, decision-making about clinical services in the NHS is evidence based. (NHSE, 1998a, p. 1)

Attention is directed to the variation between standards and levels of care, the importance of closely and systematically scrutinising areas of healthcare so that standards can be driven up and excellence and quality guaranteed to all (NHSE, 1998a).

Evidence-based practice is achieved by following a number of steps. Sackett and Rosenberg (1995) suggest:

- formulating a clear clinical question from a patient's problem
- searching the literature for relevant clinical articles
- evaluating (critically appraising) the evidence for its validity and usefulness
- implementing useful findings in practice.

Rosswurm and Larrabee (1999) have recently devised their own tried and tested model for evidence-based practice. Based on theoretical and research literature, the model follows six stages:

1. Assess the need for a change in practice
2. Link problem interventions and outcomes
3. Synthesise the best evidence
4. Design the practice change
5. Implement and evaluate the change in practice
6. Integrate and maintain the change in practice.

The overall success of the model is dependent upon the level of meticulousness maintained at each of the six stages. While most practitioners are easily able to identify and assess the need for a change in practice, the first stage in this model, the subsequent five stages of the model may pose more of a challenge. Furthermore, not all clinical problems are amenable to research (White, 1997), and it is not often that a single problem arises with a single appropriate intervention.

Research, evidence-based practice and clinical governance

Several national and international initiatives have been developed to facilitate the implementation of evidence-based practice: the NICE, the Clinical Standards Advisory Board and the Committee for Health Improvement in England, along with HSFs, are among those tasked with ensuring that clinical practice is underpinned by a substantive body of evidence. Clinical governance is part of this move to achieve a critical mass.

As previous chapters have highlighted, clinical governance is a framework into which evidence-based practice, research, clinical effectiveness and clinical supervision all fit. Proposed by the government to assure quality healthcare, it makes all healthcare professionals aware of their obligation to ensure that care given is based on the best available evidence, that it is monitored and evaluated, that quality care is demonstrated and that a public account of practice is made available to patients, healthcare providers, purchasers and professionals.

The development of clinical governance (see Chapter 2) means that organisations must make a commitment to address the organisational, cultural and methodological barriers to evidence-based practice by investing in staff development and releasing practitioners for the purpose of research. A concentrated effort is required not only for the development of evidence-based practice, but also for its associated activities, for example clinical audit and quality assurance. The links between research, evidence-based practice and clinical governance are clear, as can be seen in Figure 3.1. The cycle of evidence-based practice could just as easily be the research cycle, specifically action research, and includes the

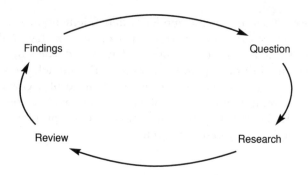

Figure 3.1   The cycle of evidence-based practice
(adapted from Sackett et al., 1996)

key aspects of accountable practice that clinical governance seeks to make explicit. So, how does evidence-based practice work in clinical practice? What follows is a more in-depth exploration of the stages of evidence-based practice, succeeded by a clinical case study demonstrating the application of theory to practice in one unit.

- *Giving care that is based on the best possible evidence*
  This entails accessing recent sources of literature, making use of existing standards and quality criteria developed from research or one's own experience, and searching for national clinical guidelines through organisations such as the NICE. This ensures that a 'combination of results from clinically relevant research, clinical expertise and patient preferences produces the best evidence for ensuring effective, individualised patient care' (Rosswurm and Larrabee, 1999, p. 317).
  Any interpretation of evidence-based practice must, however, also take into account what is meant by clinical decision-making (Walsh, 1998). The clinician is responsible for decision-making, and not all practice can be based purely on research (Sackett et al., 1996). Where research and practice are not generalisable, a consensus opinion should be sought.

- *Monitoring and evaluating care*
  This stage involves self-assessment through reflective practice and clinical supervision, as well as the development of an ongoing professional dialogue. Decisions need to be made

about who to include in the evaluation process, particular attention being paid to the role of partnerships and consumer involvement. This process of reflecting on practice enhances the development of explicit guidelines as opposed to measuring practice against implicit standards.

● *Demonstrating quality care*
Here practitioners are seeking to maintain continuous quality improvement through audit and review in a multi-disciplinary forum.

● *Public accountability of practice*
At this stage, practitioners are developing the skills of giving an account of practice. Professional practice is made open to scrutiny through the processes of reflective practice, clinical supervision, the involvement of other disciplines and the dissemination of research findings at local, national and inter-national forums.

CASE STUDY

Outlined here is a brief clinical vignette that seeks to illuminate the stages of evidence-based practice adapted to a specific clinical setting.

The first skill that clinicians need to have before evidence-based practice or clinical effectiveness can even begin is the ability to question their own practice and accept that there is possible room for improvement. Unless nurses automatically think each time they are about to be involved in clinical decision-making – am I sure that I have the best available evidence to inform me and my patient when making this decision? – evidence-based practice will receive only lip service. It is obviously not possible for a practitioner to stop and carry out a literature search before each and every clinical decision is taken. If, however, the clinical team collectively consider where they are confident that evidence-based practice is taking place, and then identify which areas they are less confident about and start to review these, a culture of constant questioning will eventually arise and evidence-based practice will be part and parcel of routine practice. This is what has happened in one unit at a large acute Trust.

The critical care unit at the Leicester Royal Infirmary has set up a quality group in order to ensure that all practice is evidence based. The staff felt that practitioners were engaging in varying clinical practices, each approaching the caring situation differently with no reference to a uniform standard. In addition, when new staff were appointed, orientation was made difficult as there were no explicit standards of practice on the unit. Staff were increasingly noticing a decline in their high standard of practice. As a result of this, volunteers were asked to form the quality group, with the remit of examining all clinical practices and working through those identified as a priority stage by stage. The group is multi-disciplinary and consists of 11 members including consultants and physiotherapists. The group takes a full day out once a month to scrutinise the relevant literature and to develop guidelines based on the best available evidence. The time-out day is funded from within the department itself and is counted towards the members' working hours. The group initially identified the clinical practices that were to be evidenced and are currently working on standards for invasive lines.

In order to pursue this, the group undertook a literature search and drew up guidelines for best evidence based on a systematic review (giving care that is based on the best possible evidence). So questioning practice and defining the problem was the first step. When preparing for a literature search, many librarians use the 'PICO' approach, that is, what is the Problem, what is the proposed Intervention, what is this being compared with (Comparison) and what is the intended Outcome? In the pursuit of evidence-based practice in nursing, nurses need to have an understanding of the different types of research and know how to appraise a published research article. They then need to be able either to take on board any suggested changes to their own practice or, where possible, influence the practice of others around them, and finally to be able to evaluate the impact of any such changes.

In the critical care unit, the guidelines, which then went out to peer review for comments to increase ownership, were put into practice and are currently (three months later) being subjected to audit (monitoring and evaluating care). An observational audit is being performed through the clinical effectiveness committee within the hospital to check whether staff are adhering to the standard, and a review date has been set (demonstrating quality care). It is envisaged that the standard will be reviewed in one year in collaboration with the quality group. The results of clinical audit could be a possible source for evidence-based practice. This is particularly true in nursing, where there are many gaps in the research evidence.

Every bed space in the unit has a copy of the guidelines, which are open to scrutiny by relatives and visitors, a copy is kept in the new staff orientation file, and the dissemination of the standards is Trust wide, copies being sent to the clinical effectiveness group and shared with the surgical directorate and recovery ward (public accountability of practice).

As yet the standards have not been published or presented at national conferences because, as we were told, 'it's what everyone does, it's nothing special'.

The difference between evidence-based practice and clinical effectiveness is that while evidence-based practice involves identifying the problem, finding the evidence to inform what to do about the problem and then implementing these findings, clinical effectiveness means taking things a step further and evaluating the impact of implementation in order to inform future care. Making practice open to public scrutiny is part of moving evidence-based practice on to clinical effectiveness. This is achieved not only through writing for publication and presenting findings at relevant venues, but also by ensuring that innovations in practice are closely monitored subsequent to their implementation.

Concluding thoughts

We have emphasised the increasing importance of research outcomes that are sensitive measures of nursing practice. It is vital that 'in the world of managed care, healthcare system variables as antecedents to outcomes demand increasing attention in nursing research' (Hoskins, 1998, p. 1). We have also identified the need for resources to be made available for the successful development of nursing research and evidence-based practice and that this is something that current policy is striving to prioritise:

National standards and effective practice need to be underpinned by a robust Nursing, Midwifery and Health Visitor evidence base. This requires investment in research and development, and in research and development expertise. (DoH, 1999a, p. 50)

To return to some of the questions posed at the beginning of this chapter, how can practitioners, educationalists, researchers, managers and policy-makers work together to actualise these ideologies? We have already indicated that if nursing is to be evidence based, 'it is necessary for a mechanism to be in place that allows and encourages them to pursue this goal' (UKCC, 1999b, p. 73).

One of the most pressing problems in addressing this goal is that of narrowing the gap that prevails between theory, practice and, more recently, research in nursing (McCaugherty,

1991; Rolfe, 1996). It is true that changes are demanding that nurses, midwives and health visitors need to be able to seek out and apply evidence, and, as such, it is essential that we improve the capability of the same to appraise and apply research findings to their practice (DoH, 1999a). Practitioners have to be empowered to identify outcomes that affect care and influence care at the clinical level. The systematic investigation of the practice of nursing is, however, a relatively new phenomenon in the nursing profession, even more so being the notion that the investigation is carried out by the practitioners themselves, that is, 'practitioner-based research' (Binnie and Titchen, 1998; Rolfe, 1998).

As much as nurses require training in research methods and data collection techniques, they also need to be re-educated to see that their nursing care can also be translated into evidence and research findings. For as Rafferty and Traynor (1999) remind us, evidence does not travel one way only (from researcher to practitioner) but is a two-way street. A number of contemporary initiatives have been developed that will tackle the issue of the practice–research gap and permit this two-way traffic, for example joint appointments and lecturer/practitioner and practitioner/researcher posts. Action research is also being more heavily utilised in order to bring occupational and organisational objectives closer together, thereby addressing the challenge of evidence-based practice (Lathlean, 1992; McSkimming, 1996).

Ensuring that the clinical standards of NSFs and NICE recommendations are implemented is a role for all nurses who have to involve themselves and take responsibility for making a difference (Freshwater, 1999). In deciding whether research findings are useful, practitioners have to evaluate whether their own personalised adaptation of the findings to a specific patient results in effective care. This means that all nurses are obliged to reflect on their practice and assess the effectiveness of the interventions that have been made, considering whether the outcomes are satisfactory, both for the nurse and for the patient. This is itself research, for the research process is a method of posing questions about nursing practice and seeking answers to them; as such, critical reflection is a critical function for any profession that claims to base its practice on evidence. The move towards establishing nursing as an evidence-based profession will be achieved through evolution rather than revolution and demands long-term vision as well as short-term goals.

Key Point Summary

▨ A constant challenge to practitioners is bringing research into practice

▨ The phrase 'evidence based' is now part of the nursing vocabulary

▨ Evidence-based practice is concerned with accountability

▨ Clinical practice must be research based

Acknowledgements

Thanks to Pauleen Pratt, Critical Care and Day Care Service Manager, Leicester Royal Infirmary, Leicester.

4

Professional Development and Clinical Supervision

Veronica Bishop

Professional development is the progress of an individual within a specific discipline or profession, which is identified by an ever-increasing understanding of, and participation in, that profession and its wider related environment. Professional development is not an activity that can occur in isolation. Its achievement is, by its very nature, a dynamic process and must involve peer review and peer support. Clinical supervision properly carried out is central to supporting professional development. This chapter briefly explores the origins of clinical supervision as it is being promoted in the nursing professions, and what it means to these professions in terms of professional development and support for the individual. The text provides some guidelines on the 'how' of its implementation and cites a case study. Some examples of how its effectiveness may be measured are discussed and further reading material is recommended.

Never have nurses had more scope, such a breadth of areas in which to work, or as much possibility for support. There are several driving forces behind this, perhaps the most influential being the publication in 1992 of the *Scope of Professional Practice* (UKCC, 1992a), which preceded the UKCC specialist practice framework and the recently published document *Fitness for Practice* (UKCC, 1999a). The *Scope of Professional Practice* provides a set of principles to guide the development and expansion of professional roles and responsibilities in nursing and midwifery. It was widely welcomed by the nursing and midwifery professions as it liberated the development of these professions from their previous reliance on task-oriented practice with vicarious accountability through doctors, towards an acceptance that activities should be limited only by the individual practitioner's knowledge and competence. The framework, which sought to facilitate more flexible practice, was intended to be advantageous for both patients' and clients' needs, and to take into account the fluctuating healthcare workforce and patterns of care. While the *Scope* document, as it became known, is seen by many to have moved nursing from its handmaiden image and traditional, more subservient way of working to specialist and advanced practitioner roles, the converse view is held by some. There are claims that *Scope* has failed to provide necessary guidance on accountability, thus leaving many nurses treading precariously on a professional highwire. There is certainly a tension between professional autonomy in nursing and the General Medical Council regulations (GMC, 1995) which state that patients are under the care of medical practitioners who have the final responsibility for those in their care.

While the debate on professional autonomy in nursing raged, other developments highlighted the need for nurses to be more flexible and to take on a wider role. These were the new deal for junior doctors (NHSME, 1991), which sought to improve the working conditions of junior doctors in line with European requirements, and the Calman Report (DoH, 1993b) which promoted shorter training for specialist doctors and a greater involvement of consultants in that training. These two documents were to have an immediate 'knock-on' effect on nurse staffing levels and nurses' responsibilities. In an increasingly litigious society, the words 'autonomy... must be fully informed' are well remembered.

Lifelong learning

How do you know what you do not know? The increase in professional knowledge, in technological advances and in drug and psychosocial therapies is too speedy and too massive for the individual practitioner wholly to assimilate it. The term 'lifelong learning' can sound exciting when one's energy level is high but very wearing if it is not. 'Lifelong learning' is an often

misused phrase, particularly when applied to training requirements rather than real learning and personal development. While
training may be essential, learning implies a deeper knowledge
base. Learning is the ability of the individual to assimilate and
consolidate what has gone before and to apply those life experiences with professional education to the benefit of both the
society within which they function and themselves. Professional
development in nursing, particularly, is dependent on learning
as well as training and cannot be achieved by academic application alone. Nursing is an interactive and dynamic discipline,
and, as such, its vital contribution to health and healthcare can
only be fully realised if nurses are willing to look beyond today's
pressing needs and focus on the wider picture.

Developments in clinical practice

Clinical practice is fundamental to nursing. Nursing may take
on other roles, but the power of nursing lies in its ability to
provide knowledgeable care, to use that knowledge to bring a
quality dimension to a period of the patient's or client's life that
would be unlikely to be achieved by a lay person. Caring is not
the prerogative of nurses: there are many people who can care,
who can be the advocate; *it is the provision of professional, knowledgeable care that must identify the nursing profession.*
   In clinical practice, the options are, as already stated, dramat-
ically increasing. The development of nurse-led services is in
part a result of the reduction in junior doctors' hours (NHSME,
1991) mentioned earlier in this chapter, and in part a need to
move from existing models of care, which are medically focused,
to provide a more patient-centred model that is responsive to
the specific needs of patients and clients. There are many
changes from traditional practice today that are either well established or are, with the new ethos of collaborative partnerships,
breaking across old barriers. Examples are the specialist roles
that have developed, such as the development of nurse-led clinics
that would once have been medically led, the collaboration of
nurses with the police in the development of nurse-led assessment services at arrests, outreach services for the socially
excluded, the NHS Direct service and nurse-led walk-in centres.

These developments owe much to the work of Pearson (1989) and his colleagues who carried out early innovative, nurse-led work in Oxford, and to the Sainsbury Family Trust who funded the first NDUs.

A critical time in this move from traditional services to more nurse-focused care delivery was the shift from charitable pump-priming funding to funding by the government in 1991. The impact of £3.2 million over five years was insignificant to the overall DoH budget, but the impact on nursing was one of a tremendous boost to morale. The subsequent DoH-funded evaluation study (Redfern et al., 1997) is important reading for those interested in the profession's development, including references on major policy initiatives that have impacted on the nursing profession over the past 10 years, not least *The Patient's Charter* (DoH, 1991a), which was the precursor of the strong user focus currently being promoted. Further important reading is the Masterclass (1998), which critiques the evaluation study and provides insight into true peer review.

The NDU initiative had a major impact on nursing services. At last there was formal recognition that nurses could and would break out of traditional moulds of task-oriented care and provide nursing that was open to change, centred on user perspectives and was willing to work in a culture of enquiry. Such units are, in many areas, still running, and they were certainly the fore-runner of the many current diverse nursing initiatives in place today. The recognition of the value of nursing, stimulated by the NDU initiative, had an enormous knock-on effect on nurses' innovations, not only in terms of clinical practice, but also in terms of formalising the newer roles such as that of the nurse practitioner/lecturer posts. These posts are often jointly funded and, as such, involve the post-holder in the tricky task of pleasing two paymasters at the same time. A platform has certainly developed that encourages collaboration between higher education and clinical areas, but it is not always a comfortable relationship, with a tension between academic standards and NHS training requirements that constantly needs adjusting.

As the profession becomes more dynamic and more complex, it is paramount that each individual nurse understands his or her own accountability and legal responsibilities. An excellent monograph by Glover (1999) on accountability is recommended to all nurses. Moving from the legal to the practical, Butterworth (1996) succinctly describes the difficulties of providing patient-centred care, and the same applies to nurse-led services. He states that the trick is to manage the tension between individuality (and burnout) and collaborative working across disciplines and management.

Developing a supportive culture: 'it's good to talk'

Much of the success of any individual in achieving his or her professional aims will depend on the vision and support of good management and careful career planning. The combined efforts of various professional nursing bodies have put clinical practice back into career advancement in nursing, a focus that the present government is more than happy to support and is indeed promoting. This change of focus, after decades of structures that gave the highest prestige to educationalists and then to managers, must be welcomed if nursing is to remain a healthcare profession.

The White Paper *The New NHS: Modern, Dependable* (DoH, 1998b), and more particularly the more recent publication *Making a Difference* (DoH, 1999a), makes it clear that the present government is committed to extending recent developments in the roles of nurses and is encouraging and supporting developments in nursing practice. *Making a Difference* is an important platform for helping the nursing professions to pursue a radical and progressive agenda (Moores, 1999). It is derived from extensive consultation across the profession and related disciplines, and brings together the aspirations of nursing within the context of the new healthcare agenda. A recent allocation of funding to appoint nurse consultants has been widely publicised in the national media, and while some media attention has mocked this innovation, it is, in the view of many, the beginning of a new era – one in which nurses will take their rightful place in the healthcare team and will be accorded remuneration reflecting the respect of society.

Career planning is rarely just a matter of having a particular talent and following it up the career ladder. Family commitments, the potential for further promotion and ease of access are some of the many issues that have to be considered within the context of what is available and what fits with one's own preferences. The joys of achieving this balance, in terms of job satisfaction and the ability to provide and deliver the quality care that students are taught to give, will be more than repaid in terms of the retention of staff, therapeutically enhanced patients and clients, and successful partnerships within the healthcare team. Historically, nursing has never appeared to be better placed to take forward a new professional status that will empower its practitioners to provide the care they are well equipped to do, taking their rightful place in society at the bedside and at the policy table. This will not be achieved by innovation alone, however well publicised. This will only be achieved, in the long term, by nursing continuing to show its reflective and dynamic abilities, and by sound research to underpin its practice (see Chapter 3).

The provision of nursing care, and the role of nursing in the multi-disciplinary healthcare team, has never been more complex, and the demands on healthcare professionals to forge multi-professional, multi-disciplinary and across-agency partnerships in the provision of that care are great. These demands cannot be met without two key constituents: first, the ability of any health professional to understand and develop from peer review, and second, the ability to communicate rather than just 'talk to' each other. Clinical supervision offers a framework that encourages, indeed is central to, these constituents. Implemented successfully, the evidence that is available indicates that a culture of caring critique, rather than a culture of blame, improves staff motivation and benefits patient care. Integral to this process comes the opportunity for the cross-fertilisation of skills, professional development and support, and communication skills – issues that are ignored at the peril of patient care.

The DoH drive to implement clinical supervision, combined with the supportive UKCC recommendation (UKCC, 1996) that it be implemented, was not accompanied by a 'recipe' on how to take it forward. There were good reasons for this, not least the desire for the profession to develop its own culture of discovery and critique: when promoting autonomy, it is counterproductive to be prescriptive. With hindsight, the profession might have found it easier to go ahead and implement clinical supervision sooner had a model been given to them; in the event, while some excellent programmes of clinical supervision are up and running, or on their way to full implementation, a plethora of misconceptions and concomitant cynicism abounds on the functions of clinical supervision. This has resulted in an apathy in some clinical localities in taking a vital mechanism forward for quality care. Some of the misconceptions derive from the term 'supervision' with its inappropriate connotations of a hierarchical system, which must be anathema to a profession seeking to be autonomous. What is important about the terminology is that the focus is on clinical practice – the heart of what nursing is about – and describes a mechanism to support the best in clinical developments (Bishop, 1998).

What is clinical supervision?

The term 'clinical supervision' stems from psychotherapy, counselling and social work but is as yet a poorly defined and developed concept in nursing. At the heart of clinical supervision is the need for peer review, staff support and public safety. Clinical supervision is about the profession entering into a relationship with itself and having the confidence from that to enter into equal partnership with other healthcare professions. This empowerment is vital if nursing is to achieve its potential in making its contribution to health and healthcare. Changes and concomitant challenges sweep across the NHS with disconcerting speed, and boundaries between disciplines and agencies are becoming more and more blurred. Quite properly, patients and their carers are moving into the centre of healthcare focus, and nurses, perhaps more than any other group of healthcare professionals, are required to meet patients' needs in as flexible a manner as possible.

Butterworth (1992), in an earlier document on clinical supervision as an emerging idea in nursing, described it as embracing a range of strategies that included preceptorship, mentorship, the supervision of qualified practice, peer review and the maintenance of professional standards. It is perhaps this breadth of constituent parts that makes the term 'clinical supervision' difficult to sum up in a neat sentence. Hart (1982) defined the activity of clinical supervision as:

> An ongoing educational process in which one person in the role of supervisor helps another in the role of supervisee to acquire appropriate professional behaviour through examination of the supervisee's professional activities.

Faugier and Butterworth (1994, p. 12) refer to clinical supervision as:

> An exchange between practising professionals to enable the development of professional skills, an opportunity to sustain and develop practice.

However, the following definition, while it does not slip easily off the tongue, is recommended. It highlights the very specific essentials of clinical supervision and is derived from discussion with fellow professionals:

> A designated interaction between two or more practitioners, within a safe/supportive environment, which enables a continuum of reflective, critical analysis of care, to ensure quality patient services. (Bishop, 1998, p. 8)

The key elements of planned, formal but confidential discussions to develop practitioners and support them in their work are embedded in this description, and it fits any model of clinical supervision used, whether it is one-to-one supervision, group supervision or supervision by remote access. It makes clear that clinical supervision is not an unplanned, unstructured activity that may take place over a quick snack in a busy canteen or staff room.

The functions of clinical supervision are well documented elsewhere (Faugier and Butterworth, 1994; Bishop, 1998). They have been adapted from work by Proctor (1992) and embrace the formative (educative and developmental) function, the restorative or debriefing and supportive function, and the normative activity of standard-setting and monitoring of those standards.

Why does nursing need clinical supervision?

The supervision of students is understood and accepted, but the culture of continuing supervision and support is new to a profession that is striving to be autonomous. It may appear to many to be contradictory to the concept of professionalism. Supervision has been statutory for midwives since 1936, and while this has, in the past, been interpreted in the main as a managerial activity with strictly hierarchical overtones, this is currently being revisited. The activity of clinical supervision as described in the definitions above, and the use of the term 'supervision' has been a part of the culture for many in mental health disciplines for decades. However, the connotations of 'big brother' and hierarchical pressure pose some difficulties for some professionals for whom the concept is new and who have not perhaps had the opportunity or made the time to investigate the term as it is being promoted in the NHS.

The emergence of clinical supervision as a central focus on the nursing agenda occurred in the 1990s, although it had been practised in some localities, and greatly valued, over many years. Developments such as NDUs, nurse-led services and further planned nursing initiatives that would involve greater autonomy than had normally been the case spearheaded new thinking for professional leaders with the responsibility of safeguarding the public as well as their members.

Demands for a workforce to be innovative, to develop new skills and constantly to update its knowledge and be responsible for its activities, as highlighted in the UKCC *Code of Professional Conduct* and the subsequent guidelines (UKCC, 1992b), carried a requirement for a facilitative framework in which professionals could flourish. A position paper distributed by the DoH (Faugier and Butterworth, 1994) set a wider train of thought into action, which was enhanced by a Delphi study (Butterworth and Bishop, 1995) highlighting responses from over 2000 skilled practitioners who supported the formal introduction of clinical supervision across all nursing specialities. Other interactive work between Trust Nurse Executives and Bishop and Butterworth (1994) established managerial support for the concept, as long as it was owned by practising nurses.

The concept of clinical supervision is not a 'flash in the pan, here today and gone tomorrow' notion as the accumulating literature (see recommended reading) demonstrates. The perceived benefits of clinical supervision are well described by Kohner (1994) and may be summed up as:

- raised professional support, staff satisfaction and well-being
- increased skill-sharing, a better information base and increased confidence
- reflective practice and increased self-awareness
- improved patient/client care.

Clinical supervision is now rooted in the document *Making a Difference* (DoH, 1999a) and will be pivotal to nurses in taking forward the government's healthcare agenda. The formalisation of clinical supervision is also supported in the UKCC document *Fitness for Practice* (1999a). If supporting excellence and valuing staff are not a priority, management at every level must, for these reasons alone, be committed to the success of clinical supervision. Clinical supervision is not a cheap option: it requires time, a budget, manpower and training.

In the longer term, preparation needs to become embedded in pre-registration nurse education, where the continuum of clinical supervision really begins. In this way clinical supervision will be expected, as a continuation of lifelong learning. As Driscoll states (2000, p. 196):

> Clinical supervision supports the clinical governance view that there is no end point in learning... clinical supervision will continually evolve, albeit slowly.

The need to change a 'macho' style of management to one of a caring critique is self-evident, particularly in the light of the dramatic current (and predicted) staff shortages in the NHS. Too many organisations have boasted to being signed up to initiatives such as Investors in People but have paid only lip service to the philosophies underpinning them. It is time that a genuine concern is demonstrated within the health service for its employees – this will then perhaps be reflected in a positive attitude to each other that demonstrates value and support. It is important to add that clinical supervision, if properly implemented, will be the greatest driver in taking forward excellence in care and assuring nursing's place at the clinical governance table (see Chapter 2). Butterworth wrote in 1998 that:

a future dream is to see any absence of clinical supervision as a curiosity; when that is so, we can be sure that its [integration] into the profession is complete. (p. 186)

How is clinical supervision carried out?

There are many different ways to take part in clinical supervision, and as long as the key elements are in place, and understood, the format is up to the individuals concerned and their agreement with their organisation. The steps outlined in Box 4.1 may serve as a helpful 'recipe' for implementation, but they are not inclusive.

Box 4.1

Negotiation with the organisation on implementation strategy

■ Is clinical supervision to be mandatory or voluntary?

■ Who in the organisation is to lead the subject?

■ What support and resources, for example a steering group, outside help, or conference and course funding, will they have?

■ How are supervisors to be selected?

■ What training is to be offered to supervisors?

■ What training is to be offered to supervisees?

■ Which staff are to be involved: qualified staff only, ancillary carers or all disciplines?

■ What mechanisms are to be used to communicate with relevant personnel?

The commitment of senior professionals to clinical supervision is without question, as is demonstrated by *Making a Difference* (DoH, 1999a). What does come into question is the necessary support, in terms of funding and personnel, to make it effective. As has been previously stated, while clinical supervision will help nurses to achieve the best level of care possible, it cannot compensate for inadequate facilities, poor management or unmotivated staff. It will, however, create a culture within which nurses can flourish if they are willing to embrace it and if management is supportive (Bishop, 1994).

Until there are enough supervisors to meet all needs, the snowball style of implementation may suit those starting out on their implementation programme (Dunn and Bishop, 1998). This means that after general information and discussion with staff, those who are appropriately qualified and would like to nominate themselves or others for the role of supervisor are put forward for training. A list may be circulated giving their names and contact numbers, and staff may approach them for supervision. It is not generally helpful to the processes of clinical supervision for supervisees to be told who to have as their supervisor, nor is it always acceptable that the supervisor be the line manager, unless the supervisee especially requests it. It is helpful to draw up a written agreement (contract) which can be used across the locality or Trust, which highlights the need for confidentiality, but also reminds users of the Code of Conduct, and any legalities stemming from that (see Box 4.2).

Box 4.2

Supervisor–supervisee relationship

- How is the supervisee allocated a supervisor?
- Is there a written contract between them setting out the expectations and ground rules?
- Is there clarity regarding confidentiality and the Code of Conduct (that is, that confidentiality cannot cover illegal or unfit conduct)?
- What will be the frequency, duration and venue of meetings?
- Are any notes of meetings to be recorded and kept?

It is important to remember that clinical supervision will, as the UKCC states, 'assist lifelong learning... throughout all registered practitioners' careers' (1996, p. 3). Clinical supervision is the formalisation of what has often been taking place informally and is about recognising that each nurse is responsible for his or her own practice and ongoing learning. The aim of clinical supervision is to enhance user and staff protection by regularly learning from experience and disseminating good practice. Staff

in caring roles need support: caring, whether it involves technical skill or personal care, is physically and emotionally wearing,
and practitioners need sustaining and time for reflection. Clinical supervision must provide this. There may be some hiccups
in its implementation as people are breaking new paths within
nursing, and this is rarely easy. It should, however, always be
remembered that clinical supervision is for the practitioners,
and in support of them and their efforts for patients and clients.

Box 4.3
Which model of clinical supervision?

- Group supervision – maximum per group?
- One-to-one supervision
- Paired supervision (two supervisees per session)
- Electronic supervision, for example email or telephone and so on.

Discussion needs to be held as to which model of clinical
supervision will best suit those considering its implementation.
Some people benefit from group supervision, others prefer one-
to-one exchanges. Time, cost and available expertise are considerations here (see Box 4.3).

Having stressed that clinical supervision is about lifelong
learning and skill-sharing, it is important for both supervisors (who
should be receiving clinical supervision as well as giving it) and
supervisees to get the most out of the process. People often say
that the hardest part of clinical supervision is the very first meeting.
How do you start? Remember that the agenda is set for the practitioners – it is their space and time. Plan a flexible set of issues;
discussions usually start by centring on the supervisee's case load
or on a specific patient. As the rapport with the supervisor
develops, so too will the depth and breadth of discussions change.

While clinical supervision is not a replacement for appraisal
mechanisms, it should provide the opportunity for individuals
to consider the wider context of healthcare and their desired
place within that. Some people find it helpful to list objectives
to be met by the next supervisory meeting; others do not, as
this in some ways mimics appraisal and restricts the potential

for spontaneous learning. What is essential is that, whatever agenda develops, the users of clinical supervision must root it in clinical practice. This will not, as various writers have agreed, occur overnight. Much will depend on the experiences of the supervisor and supervisee and their ongoing relationship. Skill is needed by both parties.

CASE STUDY

Clinical supervision gets started

The Ravensbourne NHS Trust in urban Kent provides community services for a population of over 275,000. These services embrace learning disabilities, health visiting, district nursing, dental and dietetics, as well as chiropody, speech and language therapy, physiotherapy and occupational therapy, the qualified and ancillary staff totalling just over 1000 individuals. This case study gives a step-by-step description of how clinical supervision is being introduced across the Trust, to all qualified and unqualified staff who care for patients and clients.

Step 1: Raising the issue

In 1997 an initial questionnaire was circulated during a nurses' staff meeting (to ensure a high response rate) with the aim of eliciting the level of knowledge of and interest in clinical supervision. Seventy-seven per cent of those approached responded. The responses indicated a high level of interest in clinical supervision, but a significant number of respondents cited anxieties about the structure and nature of the process. A core group of 20 senior nurses was encouraged to attend a three-day clinical supervision skills workshop with an external trainer in order to train them to be supervisors. From the comments made at a later conference, this workshop was particularly successful, the key reason being the enthusiasm and expertise of the external trainer. These supervisors went on to give and receive supervision and were later joined by 18 more supervisees.

This approach could be criticised for possibly giving the erroneous impression that clinical supervisors must be senior (thus making clinical supervision a hierarchical activity) to more junior staff. Nonetheless, this activity put clinical supervision on the Trust agenda, and selected staff were involved in piloting clinical supervision. A feasibility study was undertaken, in collaboration with staff from the Division of Nursing, Kings College, which explored users' satisfaction with clinical supervision. This was completed in January 1999, the subsequent report of the study recommending the Trust-wide implementation of clinical supervision for nurses. The appointment of a new chief executive then brought to the Trust a renewed energy in implementation strategies.

Step 2: Making the strategy reality

The chief executive had, in a previous senior nurse post, employed a successful strategy to implement clinical supervision. Not wishing to lose any further momentum from the initial efforts in Ravensbourne, she authorised a one-day conference to put clinical supervision into high profile, stressing that it was Trust policy for all clinical staff, in all disciplines, both qualified and unqualified, to participate in clinical supervision. An interim policy statement was issued at the onset of the new millennium recording that the Ravensbourne Trust believed clinical supervision to be critical to achieving and maintaining continuous improved quality healthcare, and to be integral to clinical governance. An experienced external facilitator (the author), in collaboration with key members of staff, devised the format for the conference, a pre-conference pack being designed that would provide relevant material to participants. Most importantly, speakers reflecting some of the various disciplines working within the Trust were drawn into a major part of the programme to discuss their experiences and views on clinical supervision. Participation was further ensured by the involvement of all attendees in smaller group work.

Step 3: Individual voices, shared experiences

The aim of the conference was to raise awareness and understanding of the concept of clinical supervision and its application to practitioners in the Trust. Participants were also to agree three key issues that would be embedded in the Trust's clinical supervision policy and to identify three personal objectives in becoming actively involved in the process. The keynote speaker laid the ground for later presentations, drawing from a national perspective and highlighting what clinical supervision is and what it is not. She stressed the enormous power of clinical supervision, if it is implemented effectively, and demystified some of the perceptions of it being a management tool.

The speakers from within the Trust brought very different perspectives to the conference, all making an important contribution for their peers to mull over. The first, a tissue viability specialist nurse, spoke enthusiastically of the training workshop she had attended, and she has since become a supervisor to three members of staff. She sees clinical supervision as a multi-disciplinary activity that supports creative solutions and lowers the stress level, now taking for granted its inclusion in the service culture. The second speaker, a child psychologist in the learning disability services, described a slightly different model of clinical supervision in that the process took her from novice to expert, becoming less and less hierarchical as her skills developed. Having been through several modes of clinical supervision, mandatory for her in her role as a registered psychologist, she illustrated three examples of supervision:

- *type 1* – disorganised, unfocused, easily cancelled and lacking any real commitment, which left her feeling frustrated and unsupported

- *type 2* – 'control freak' supervision, the supervisor taking a controlling and prescriptive role, leaving her demoralised

- *type 3* – symbiotic, with a balance between clinical and academic work, and time to think through previous work and to plan ahead. Mistakes were acknowledged and learned from.

This speaker stressed that the supervisor is for her not a 'solutions' person but more of a brainstorming companion.

The newly qualified community nurse valued his clinical supervision highly, finding that it offered shared learning if the power imbalance between the supervisee and supervisor was sensitively handled. An emphasis was laid here on the need to book meetings well in advance and to draw up ground rules between the supervisor and recipients. A diabetes specialist nurse queried what made an expert, stressing the value of the individual and his or her 'lived' knowledge. She valued clinical supervision in that it gave her time to reflect and to feel a part of the 'organisational unity'.

A senior specialist speech and language therapist described her very isolated work patterns and the mechanism that she had developed to maintain team membership and peer review. She had adopted a very dynamic approach, mixing and matching available resources and people for her needs, which had so far successfully prevented her 'tearing my hair out'. A nursing home liaison nurse voiced some scepticism as to the organisational goodwill towards clinical supervision in terms of the time needed to sustain its implementation and the ability of nurses in particular to break the 'care and cope' mentality attributed to them.

The final speaker had confessed in her abstract in the conference pack that she had filled in the reply slip to attend the conference and inadvertently ticked a box saying that she would speak! This very honest team leader in a multi-disciplinary community care team is a supervisor but has not received any supervision herself. Her cry of 'my biggest problem at work is not having enough time to achieve all that I want to achieve!' must be familiar to most of us, but her admission that we must not get blinded by our own perceptions touches at the heart of our need for clinical supervision.

Step 4: Developing a shared agenda

The group work at this conference focused on the identification of three issues that the attendees wished to be addressed at the top management, policy-making level in the Trust. This group activity met several objectives apart from the input to executive decision-making, the main ones being:

- a chance for people to network in a multi-disciplinary forum

- meeting people they had not met before: group members were allocated by the organisers, thus excluding the possibility of cliques forming

- an opportunity better to understand the issues involved in clinical supervision and thus dispose of some of the myths surrounding it.

The level of enthusiasm was generally high, the atmosphere being one of 'can do' rather than 'if only'. More clinical supervision meetings were called for, to be highlighted by road shows and in-house marketing, training and education. A strong view of the majority of participants was that clinical supervision should be compulsory (and stated in the employing contract) within the Trust, as long as training was *accessible,* and clinical supervision should be included in induction courses *for all staff.* A focus of central coordination was sought that would establish procedures to determine the allocation of supervisors and the limit on the number of supervisees to be allocated to one supervisor, as well as to organise a directory of supervisors and their specific areas of clinical interest and expertise. Issues to be addressed, such as agreements between supervisees and their supervisors, ground rules and confidentiality, were stressed, as was the need for protected time and resources. It was the strongly held view of the participants that the successful implementation and uptake of clinical supervision would depend on an acknowledgement from top management of the priority accorded to it within the Trust.

The three key policy issues identified with the agreement of all participants were:

- key people to be identified to take clinical supervision forward across the Trust, to coordinate activities and to create a directory for access to supervisors

- clinical supervision training to be available to all clinical staff, both qualified and ancillary

- protected time for clinical supervision.

In her commitment to supporting staff in achieving excellence in care, the chief executive concluded the conference by signing up to these issues, the agreed strategy to be revisited in a similar forum within a year.

The author is very grateful to all participants at the conference; their generosity and openness were remarkable and bode well for the success of their implementation programme. Sincere thanks also go to the chief executive who agreed to the proceedings being used as a case study for this chapter.

Audit and evaluation of clinical supervision

The demand for evidence-based activity is one placing a great deal of pressure on all healthcare professionals, and rightly so. In nursing, however, the challenge is emphasised still further, if only for the reason that nursing care is all pervasive and rarely the result of a single intervention in a totally controlled environment.

Audit should not be confused with evaluation. Audit is concerned with checking or verifying activities, and in clinical supervision an audit may be useful to check the uptake of clinical supervision by records of sessions, notes of cancellations and so on. The evaluation of its effectiveness will be enhanced by audit measures, but these will provide only numerical rather than descriptive information.

The subject of evaluating clinical supervision for nurses and health visitors was addressed in a major study funded by the DoH and undertaken at Manchester University (Butterworth et al., 1996a). Despite the vast amount of anecdotal evidence that clinical supervision benefits individuals and their practice, the instruments used to measure any change in staff well-being in this multi-site study demonstrated little of statistical significance (Butterworth et al., 1996a). What was clearly needed was the development of a more sensitive instrument, one that would be well validated and provide quantitative information. Manchester University has duly undertaken this task, and the Manchester Clinical Supervision Scale, which was launched by the Chief Nursing Officer for England in January 2000 is now available on a consultancy basis (Winstanley, 1999).

From the data generated by a national database, Winstanley has found that nursing staff report improved care and skills, as well as increased job satisfaction, as a result of effective clinical supervision. The data collected so far indicate that group sessions are more effective than one-to-one sessions, and sessions away from the workplace are more effective. Longer sessions, that is lasting for at least one hour, held at least monthly are more effective than shorter, less frequent meetings. The most important advice to remember, when faced with the difficulty of finding evidence to support clinical supervision (or any other activity), is that an absence of evidence does not necessarily equate with evidence of absence.

Conclusion

To have a passion for nursing is to embrace the challenge of changing healthcare needs and to consider how to develop strategies to support the best of nursing care. Changing health needs and patterns of care offer a unique opportunity for the nurse to offer care that is sensitive to patients' cultural needs and really to make care 'user centred' and less fragmented than is currently the case. This chapter has sought to provide a brief insight into how nursing arrived where it is today in terms of a developing profession, and to highlight key issues and opportunities for those healthcare staff who want to achieve their individual professional potential and contribute effectively to the national healthcare programme.

Key Point Summary

- Professional development is a dynamic process
- Professional development depends on a sound knowledge base
- How do you know what you do not know?
- Professional development must involve peer support and critique

---

Suggested further reading

Jassper, M., Arolfe, G. and Chambers, N. (2000) *Critical Reflection for Nursing and the Helping Professions: A User's Guide.* London: Macmillan.
Tschudin, V. (1999) *Nurses Matter.* London: Macmillan.

5

Developing Clinical Practice

Veronica Bishop and Irene Scott

This chapter considers the views obtained from a series of focus groups that aimed to identify the inhibitors and facilitators encountered in developing clinical practice. What then are the enablers and inhibitors of a good learning experience, which is key to the advancement of sustained practice development? Key elements identified by the 60 group participants addressed organisational, professional and attitudinal issues, and these are discussed within the context of the debates held. While the views stated must be acknowledged as deriving from a self-selected group within a specific region, they have a wider resonance and are applicable across the UK, posing challenges for the future of nursing and its position in healthcare. Positive activities that can be promoted to support, enable and facilitate innovative, sustainable and effective practices are described. We are writing at an exciting time in healthcare development, when nursing must rise to the challenge of influencing and driving the change agenda.

Strategies for developing clinical practice must not be advanced in a vacuum; in other words, policy must be informed by practitioners and, just as importantly, practitioners must occasionally stand back and examine their local options and possibilities. The role of research needs to be taken into account within the debate on developing clinical practice, and consideration must be given to how best academia can support clinical practice. The provision of expert clinical care is a dynamic process and, as such, must be constantly questioned, evaluated and adapted to suit each individual and each situation. To achieve this, health-care professionals must develop an open approach to learning, one that, although critical, is able to appreciate new ideas and test them knowledgeably. What then constitutes a good learning experience, an environment in which critique and access to information are second nature? And what organisational and professional frameworks can support this 'can do, have a go' culture?

The views of practitioners were sought through focus groups on these issues, which are central to high-quality patient care and to the well-being of healthcare staff striving to provide excellence. The value of holding focus groups is twofold: local issues generally translate into the wider arena, and lessons may be learnt that have a far wider application than just the parochial. Importantly, stake-holders, these being practitioners, have a voice and are heard within a context that has the potential to be productive and produce very positive results. This type of approach offers participants the opportunity to recognise that many others share their feelings, beliefs and views, and therefore creates licence to articulate and participate in a relatively 'safe' environment.

It is the strongly held view of the authors, and one that is shared by many leaders within the nursing professions (Bishop, 1999; Johnston, 1999b; Moores, 1999; Pearson, A., 1998; Pearson, M., 2000; Stevens, 1997), that the power of nursing lies in its clinical expertise and development, and the underpinning of that development by research evidence. The term 'research' is off-putting to some people, who would prefer to develop an expertise, or learn a way of carrying out a task, and stick with it if it appears to work. There is much to be said for that – as long as the practitioner has considered the effectiveness of his or her practice.

In a nutshell, however, how do you know what you do not know? Experience is a great teacher, but the learning is only as broad as the individual's understanding and must, by definition, be coloured by his or her own values and judgements. Properly conducted research offers the opportunity to reach beyond the experience, interpretation and understanding of one individual in order to obtain a collective judgement that is, generally speaking, derived from parameters or variables that are as controlled as possible. This can be quite difficult when researching issues that relate to people, so there is much debate, particularly in the nursing professions, on what constitutes 'good' research.

It is not the remit of this book to develop this argument further, but suggested reading for those who would like to pursue the subject is listed at the end of the chapter. What is really important for our purposes is to support best clinical practice and those nurses involved in the provision of patient care. This can only be achieved by espousing the philosophy that clinical practice is always approached with a questioning attitude and with an (albeit tempered) enthusiasm to recognise the benefits and accept a change from accepted or traditional practices.

Make the time – question practices

As autonomous practitioners, it is essential that nurses review their practices and keep up to date. The opportunity is, however, rarely offered to practitioners to stand back and examine, with their peers, how best to take this development forward. Within the confines of a busy day, conflicting hierarchies and 'getting a life' outside work can present quite a challenge. It is a challenge, however, that must be accepted, and it is up to each practitioner to work out how best to do this. The most helpful and legitimate method is through clinical supervision (see Chapter 4), through reading professional journals and by attending conferences on an individual speciality. Accessing research conferences or seminars in a specific area is another option, and will encourage a wider perspective.

In considering how to take a wider perspective and gain the views of more people who can easily and quickly be interviewed individually, it is helpful to consider the use of focus groups. These afford a free-flowing discussion on specific topics, requiring a facilitator or researcher to maintain the theme or focus while encouraging debate. Focus groups, while not new as a means of collecting information, have recently come into vogue through their much publicised use by the UK government. The joint participation of the facilitator and the participants affords a working partnership that has the potential to achieve goals consensus; thus a degree of compliance may be expected to support any implementation strategy. Brainstorming techniques may be used to explore existing and/or ideal situations, and critical incidences can be examined to identify current barriers to achieving the shared vision. The advantages of obtaining a great deal of information from a group of appropriately selected participants within a short time must, however, be weighed against the possibility of stronger voices or opinions predominating. It is here particularly that the skill of the researcher/facilitator is most needed to maintain a balance and keep a focus on the desired outcome.

There is some dispute concerning the validity of focus groups as a research tool (Breakwell et al., 1995), but, used in conjunction with other research instruments, they may yield important data. For the purposes of the activity described here, they met the set purpose of a well-targeted and designed meeting from which barriers to changing clinical practice, and mechanisms that exist to support change, were identified in a major city.

The activities described in this chapter are easily replicated elsewhere, and, given one or two skilled facilitators, the benefits of focus groups can be many. They provide 'time out', they offer the opportunity for airing views that may otherwise fester and create dissonance in a wider but more vulnerable arena, and they stimulate critical thinking, which can be put to very positive use in any locality. What is essential if the groups or workshops are to be effective is the agreement of an outcome, for example a publication or managerial commitment.

CASE STUDY

An invitation from two professors of nursing was sent to every Trust in a major city to send as many qualified clinically based nurses as possible, from all clinical localities, both primary and secondary, to attend a series of focus groups (Figure 5.1). These groups would, through group participation, obtain views on the inhibitors and the facilitators for developing clinical practice, and identify what is good and not so good about the present learning process.

Sixty nurses and midwives from the acute and community services were interested and welcomed the opportunity to participate. Their grades ranged from student nurse to senior manager and specialist nurse, the ratio of male to female being within normal UK parameters at about 1:9. The participants, many of whom had never met before, came from a large inner city with a nursing workforce in excess of 5,000. Their host organisations each held their own values and therefore had unique leadership styles and organisational goals. It is therefore important to recog-

Challenges to Developing Clinical Practice

This could be your unique opportunity to influence how nurses of the future influence, undertake and implement the development of clinical practice.

We are looking for nurses from all grades and specialities to give their views through focus group participation in order to enable the gathering of enough data to enable nursing development in Leicester to be built on evidence.

It is our intention to hold a focus group to:

● explore what the inhibitors to developing clinical practice are

● discover what the facilitators of developing clinical practice are

● outline what is good or bad in the learning process

● identify possible case studies.

The findings will be written up, disseminated and later transcribed into a chapter in a book – an acknowledgement of contribution will be made!

Date: ....

Time: 0900–1200

LUNCH WILL BE PROVIDED

Interested? We would love to hear from you.

Please contact: ....

Figure 5.1   Case study invitation

nise both the limitations and the richness of the data obtained through discussion. It is also of value to note that the disparity of the organisations and the excellent facilitation enabled an unusual opportunity to share thoughts in a safe environment.

The age range of the participants was wide, ranging from early twenties to late fifties, thus providing a breadth of life experience and professional expertise. Participants were divided into four randomly selected groups, preventing friends staying together and offering the opportunity to network. Most importantly for our purposes, this strategy facilitated discussions around a continuum of patient care across the primary and secondary care sectors.

In circumstances such as these, it is essential first to undertake a brief exercise to enable participants to feel comfortable and at ease with people whom they may not have previously met or whom they may regard as their seniors. To this end, the facilitators undertook an introduction exercise including expectations of the focus group work. It is essential at this stage to gain participants' willingness to be open and free with their thoughts, with a strong recognition that direct comments will not be attributed to named individuals. The focus groups aimed to blend the care sectors' various experiences, not only facilitating dialogue for the purposes of this event, but also generating future working relationships across the sector boundaries. The essence of the success of this type of event is to create an environment that is safe, productive and fun. The collected data from the event clearly demonstrated the success of the facilitators.

Developing clinical practice

What then, in the view of our 60 participants, were the main enablers of and inhibitors to developing clinical practice? The groups were invited to consider this, analyses of the data obtained indicating that the inhibitors fell within three sub-groups. A strong and continual focus highlighted feelings of disempowerment from the sheer speed of change within the NHS, the fact that changes were introduced without pause or, so it seemed to many, without a due consideration of what had gone before, a lack of context and organisational memory giving many a feeling of being out of control.

'Progress' can feel like being an anonymous cog in some great wheel and render progress as a very empty promise. The dangers of this are discussed by the management guru Charles Handy (1994), and effective healthcare depends, as does good business, on staff being and *feeling* involved in the aims of their organisation, at local and national level. This seemingly empty promise of progress can be resolved, and while the groups involved in this case study had suffered somewhat from the unprecedented speed of change, imposed by two apparently differing governments, both of whom used the NHS as a political football, the participants had a strong view on how, within existing organisations, changes could be made for improved working and an increased quality of care. These changes did not depend on a 'blue skies' scenario, but they did assume a shared agenda and therefore shared values for improvement from the top of any organisation down to the grass roots.

The key characteristics, or headings, of the issues discussed may be listed as:

- organisational/managerial

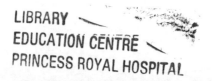

- professional/leadership

- attitudinal.

Organisational and managerial issues: sharing ownership and values

The discussions that generated the data in Box 5.1 below demonstrated a vivid sense of powerlessness in the groups, which may be seen as somewhat surprising given that they comprised highly articulate, self-selected nurses, midwives and health visitors, many of whom were in a relatively senior position. There was a strong view within all the groups that nurses' work was not highly valued, either in the NHS or generally, by the UK public. This lack of value was, in the view of the groups, indicative of society's valuing of 'women's work', which they perceived as generally low and which they saw as being reflected in managers' attitudes across the healthcare services. This is a view that is discussed in more detail elsewhere (Robinson, 1992; Salvage, 1992) and one that the newcomer to nursing in the UK may find helpful to consider further.

Some members of the groups were of the view that they were becoming deskilled as a result of skill mix, which they saw as a euphemism for grade mix. Staff shortages and the reduction in junior doctors' hours were cited as drivers for a blurring of professional boundaries in a way that was not necessarily detrimental to patient care but certainly devalued professional nursing as its workforce was used to plug any deficit. Despite their skill and commitment to the healthcare agenda, the participants suffered from a lack of clarity in terms of their value to service provision.

All this may sound somewhat depressing and deter the reader from pursuing the debate and discussion further, but this should not be the case. What the data highlight is the need for support through change, which is fully addressed in Chapter 1. The real opportunity for nursing lies in its recognition and understanding of the influential factors in the need for change. Embrace change rather than have it done to you! It is central to change to understand the opposing forces that arise from within a group and from its host organisation. As a general rule, most employees want to share the aims and goals of their employers, and it is a singularly foolish employer who does not seek to maximise staff input. The NHSME document (1993, p. 17) particularly emphasised the importance of teamworking saying:

> The best and most cost-effective outcomes for patients and clients are achieved when professionals work together, learn together, engage in clinical audit of outcomes together, and generate innovation to ensure progress in practice and service.

While this statement was particularly aimed at teamworking in health and social care, the tenets expressed have now been adopted by the current government to serve any organisation at any level. Poor communication from either 'side' of the employment fence is usually at the seat of most antagonisms within any organisation. The larger the organisation, and thus a greater reduction in close, two-way communication, the greater the opportunity for discord. Research (West and Poulton, 1997; West, 1999) has shown that the greatest barriers to effective teamwork and communication are the organisational context and the lack of appropriate support structures and integration systems. The overall picture to be drawn from the comments received in the focus groups is one of a body of skilled professionals who have not been able to carve out a clear identity for themselves.

It is essential to consider how to maximise those skills for the benefit of the health services and the well-being of the professional. A workforce that feels disempowered *is* disempowered. A simple demonstration of this was indicated by the fact that the participants found the language in government missives and technical initiatives such as audit and complaints procedures difficult to understand; thus these appear to bypass the very people whom they affect. This was clearly recognised by the groups in this case study, and some strong mechanisms, highlighted in Box 5.1, are suggested to enhance organisational activity and personal achievements within that sphere.

To take forward the issues raised in Box 5.1 would mean dropping a great deal of the old baggage that comes with traditional nursing attitudes. That is, the old culture of 'them and us', 'them' being anyone not involved in clinical care perceived as an opposing force. Was this a very self-motivated body of nurses and midwives, or were they voicing a view that is developing across the whole of nursing in the UK? Self-critique must be seen as a sign of a maturing profession.

This is to be welcomed as it underpins the philosophy of the consultation document *A Health Service of All Talents: Developing the NHS Workforce* (DoH, 2000b), which proposes wide-ranging and radical changes to the way in which NHS staff are educated and trained. The theme, however, is simple – to support excellence in care. This document is to be welcomed in enabling a change in culture as identified by the group.

While management 'bashing' is common practice in most organisations, not least the NHS, the groups did not indulge themselves here, demonstrating professional maturity and a recognition on their part of the difficulties faced by managers. Instead, participants sought to identify, in a positive manner, ways whereby management at every level could

Box 5.1

Organisational and managerial issues to enhance achievement

Positive

- Organisational openness
- Stability within a change culture
- Matching of workload to meet staff level
- Long-term planning
- Allowing staff ownership of decisions
- Saying 'thank you' and valuing staff
- Policy initiatives being stated in user-friendly language
- Seeking comments or suggestions from staff
- Supporting management

Negative

- Lack of shared vision between management and clinical staff
- Crisis planning
- Poor multi-disciplinary working
- Blurring of professional boundaries, without accountability
- Skill mix/grade mix; lack of power and autonomy
- No staff support

maximise the efforts of their staff without increasing the stress level. There was some sympathy for the pressure under which NHS organisations have been put for some years, not least with a new government anxious to prove that it could match its previous expertise as a challenging shadow Parliament of many years, by effecting significant change for the better.

Many of the focus group members felt that they would be able to offer more support than was currently the case if their organisations were more open about the pressure they were suffering and included them in decision-making. It was the perception of the some members of the groups that management lurched from crisis to crisis – using an Elastoplast to fix a running sore, rather than accessing views from the main workforce to contribute to an agreed overall policy. Others in the groups, however, enjoyed very open and receptive management styles, and those in managerial roles actively sought to create an open style of governance with clear goals and shared core values.

Sharing ownership

The groups agreed that the sharing of standards set within Trusts and nationally was essential. The opportunity to share best practice is fundamental to progress in excellent care; not to have this opportunity can create feelings of vulnerability in matters such as litigation and risk management. While a 'blame-free' culture is being fostered in the NHS, the role of the practitioner in advancing practice may be one of discomfort if he or she has not been involved in organisational policies for care provision.

Box 5.2 identifies the positive and negative aspects of clinical innovation and audit. Participants viewed staff appraisals and staff support systems as being integral to supporting change management, and wanted the opportunity to reflect on complaints and audit reviews. The current drive to involve users was welcomed, the move to identify closer links here being seen as overdue and to be welcomed. It was, however, thought prudent to evaluate the effectiveness of any mechanism used to achieve this in order to prevent user involvement becoming tokenistic.

There are many good examples of innovation in this area, one of particular interest to this group being the approach taken by the Leicester Royal Infirmary during its radical change management programme, which spanned four years. At the beginning of the programme, they randomly selected over 50 complainants from their closed complaints files and invited

---

Box 5.2

Positive and negative aspects of clinical innovation and auditing

Positive
- Shared change management principles
- Regular staff appraisal
- Involvement with audit
- Accessible information technology (IT)
- Support mechanisms for staff, for example clinical supervision
- Shared information
- Patient/user involvement
- Learning from good and bad practices

Negative
- Poor IT resources
- Lack of IT training
- Poor closing of audit 'loop'
- Poor staff support mechanisms
- Non-sharing culture
- No time to reflect

them to an open evening at which the aspirations of the Trust were shared. Participants were encouraged to form a patients' council, which was later to become a highly challenging organisation. The expertise of this group was accessed to challenge the Trust in its vision and its organisation of services and care. Fears that the council could become institutionalised were allayed following an independent audit and evaluation of its work. As the organisation matured, so did the council, and in time council members agreed to disband and reform into more localised groups. This is mirrored in another city, where patient-focused participation schemes have been actively employed in specific areas of clinical practice.

Professional issues

Several members of the groups felt that nursing had 'lost its way', many others considering nursing to be a quasi-profession in that it has little autonomy, less apparent power and a history that does not reflect the established components of a profession, such as law or medicine. It was mooted that nursing was suffered a lifelong attitude that had been developed 'below stairs', had not yet cultivated the right culture to reflect any progress in political and clinical terms and thus had not yet earned the right to be called a profession. The question 'does nursing continue to borrow an image of professionalism that may be outdated or inappropriate?' may well be asked. Rather than looking to archaic versions of professionalism, nursing should perhaps unapologetically carve its own niche and have the courage of the newly launched 'Internet millionaires'. Nursing has the education; it has the skills; it has a huge demand for these attributes – it should take the power and use it to demonstrate that today's professionals are collaborative, wide-serving individuals who can adapt their advanced education to serve the population in meeting its healthcare needs.

One of the reasons why writing the above statement is far easier than living it is that nursing is often very unspecific, too little work as yet having been carried out on the value and effectiveness of nurses' interventions. These interventions must include what are often perceived to be 'soft' activities, which are often impossible, with the instruments currently available, to isolate from other influences. The theory of a therapeutic environment, while not new (it was discussed long ago by Hippocrates (460–370 BC)) and albeit anecdotally is well established, does not possess substantive data to support its relevance to improved health. The understandable, but very limiting, preference for randomised controlled trials as the gold standard for measuring effectiveness has done nursing few favours. Nor has nursing yet developed a strong enough voice on different methodologies to effectively counter-balance the current, medically dominated research domain. Littlewood (1989) notes the crucial role of nursing in assessing and managing chronic illness, disability and the health problems of particularly the elderly, for which the quick-fix medical model is inappropriate. In essence, nurses have the opportunity to have a greater impact on the quality of life. The groups within this case study considered it essential that methods of audit highlighting nursing interventions should be developed; as yet, there are scant quantitative data that demonstrate their effectiveness.

Continuing with the theme of research, all four groups considered that nurses could not readily introduce research-based changes until the profession recognised its strengths and abilities. To do so was often fraught with insurmountable difficulties and anecdotes were provided that clearly illustrated the ensuing 'hoo-ha' when attempting to change outdated practices, particularly those long established by medical colleagues. This highlighted for many participants the lack of a shared, multi-disciplinary vision for healthcare, which was sometimes exacerbated by conflicts between managers and clinical staff. Before the ink is dry on this book, the implementation of clinical governance (see Chapter 2) should have gained momentum and offered a clear opportunitiy for nurses and nursing to influence research-based care.

The four groups in the study were very much in unison when asked to identify those elements in their organisations which did, or could, facilitate the development of innovative clinical practices and those which would prevent this. These are shown in Box 5.3.

The central message that predominated in this theme was the need to keep skilled nurses in clinical practice and to demonstrate their value by supporting their decision to stay in clinical practice. This could be facilitated by the development of career opportunities in line with changing clinical practice, and by a real commitment to more flexible working patterns, on the part of not only managers, but also full-time colleagues. Each individual could contribute to a valuing society – maybe something as simple as saying 'thank you' to colleagues. The key message here from the focus groups was to stress the concept of staff caring for each other. This was seen as essential if nursing was to move forward in a collegiate and successful way. Valuing staff is not just the province of managers, although appreciation from this quarter is always welcome. Areas in which care or staff motivation was at a higher level than the local norm should be highlighted and the vision of excellence shared.

Opportunities recognised by the groups that are available, and which should be grasped to strengthen nursing and its contribution to healthcare, were developments in audit, with concomitant research and development 'back-up'. The need to be able to access easily information on evidence-based practice was stressed, as was the desire for a greater

---

Box 5.3
Professional issues in clinical innovation

Positive

- Clear professional leadership
- Good use of resources, for instance link nurses and communication networks
- Saying 'thank you'
- Good mentorship/support mechanisms, for example clinical supervision
- Time to develop, evaluate and reassess
- Identification of local academic resources
- Development of academic/ clinical roles
- Multi-disciplinary learning/ sharing

Negative

- Lack of unity in nursing
- Lack of professional power, poor discipline and tendency to play safe
- Non-sharing culture
- Unsupportive environment
- Acceptance of transferability of skills without accountability
- Poor academic links with practice areas

---

accessibility of research and development programmes for nurses, not necessarily leading to degrees or diplomas. What was seen by many participants as a key to success in developing practice was the need to demystify some aspects of research and provide an opportunity for nurses to become comfortable with reading and utilising research findings. It was universally agreed by all the groups that there is an urgent need for the profession to change its current culture, from one that is often unquestioning to one of self-critique and professional growth.

Attitudes

Members of the groups considered that attitudes are, in many ways, contagious and thought that nursing must take some of the blame for the longstanding and still dominant 'blame' culture that is prevalent in the NHS. Box 5.4 highlights the changes in attitude that, in the views of the participants, are needed in order to break away from old and negative patterns of behaviour.

Box 5.4

Attitudinal issues in clinical innovation

- Positive attitude – putting words into action
- Owning your problems
- Challenging unfavourable behaviours
- Spending less time moaning – focus on doing
- Continuous improvement – not unevaluated change
- Lifelong learning
- Professional openness – it is OK to make a mistake and OK to challenge it
- Giving and receiving feedback

To change the current predominant culture, the groups agreed that the profession must take responsibility for its own learning, its own actions and the concomitant accountability. Participants accepted that this new ethos of sharing and critique would not occur overnight but strongly desired a mechanism to support change. In identifying aspects of lifelong training among themselves, they highlighted the issues in Box 5.5 as being essential.

Supported by the need to develop and maintain a professional portfolio (UKCC, 1994), the groups demonstrated a keen understanding of the value of lifelong learning and sought to encourage a culture in which challenge and user involvement underpinned developments in clinical care. Many of these elements are, in the view of the groups, applicable across the multi-disciplinary board rather than being merely a problem within nursing.

What then, in the view of the groups, made learning a valuable and effective experience? Box 5.6 highlights the key categories identified by

---

Box 5.5

Lifelong learning

- Sharing information
- Learning from good and bad practices
- Patient focus and involvement of users

Box 5.6

Key categories of factors affecting learning

- Culture
- Environment
- Motivation
- Resources/equipment
- Time
- Expectations
- Initiative

- Commitment
- Attitude
- Necessity
- Structure
- Finance
- Support
- Non-judgemental

---

the groups when they were asked to consider the enablers and inhibitors of good learning.

The groups chose to select three specific issues to discuss in greater detail as these were considered to be fundamental:

- professional/cultural
- organisation
- attitudes.

Professional/cultural issues

The culture of a profession or organisation was seen to be a fundamental factor that could enable or disable learning, in either the clinical or the academic environment. Culture was seen to drive expectations and influence desire and effect, and was considered to create results that were potentially both positive and negative, as indicated in Box 5.7. The culture within an organisation will largely depend on those in positions of power or in management or leadership roles, and on whether there is an inclusive or an exclusive approach to achieving vision and goals. While there were five main Trusts represented in this discussion, and many more professional groups, there was a clear agreement that even where subcultures existed, there were many common themes emanating from all the organisations.

There was a clear articulation of the events of recent years that were perceived to demonstrate a limited cultural change. The introduction of 'clinical grading', for example, was seen to have strengthened the system of hierarchy, which had been generated years previously, and which, for some inexplicable reason, nurses appeared to feel the need to hang on

Box 5.7

Professional/cultural issues influencing learning

Positive

- Encouragement
- Ability and opportunity to feed back experience
- Recognition that time taken out to learn is acceptable and necessary
- Peer pressure and support
- Academic expectations can support access to higher learning
- 'Custom and practice' *can* offer some good learning options – 'don't throw the baby out with the bath water!'
- Acceptance of failing
- Challenging – creating a desire to pursue further development
- Time spent on development is recognised as valuable

Negative

- Strength of hierarchy – clinical grading
- Negative attitudes to those returning from longer periods of study leave
- Peer pressure to keep up with academic success
- Academic expectations can generate a feeling of inadequacy
- 'Custom and practice' is often bad practice passed on from one generation to another, without evidence
- It is not OK to be seen to fail
- Challenge is often viewed as a threat, having a negative affect particularly on undergraduate students who are expected to question practice

to. Interestingly, while it was recognised that there was now a positive move to reduce the nursing hierarchy in organisations, this was seen as being replaced by an academic hierarchy, by a need for nurses to demonstrate their ability to achieve not only in practice, but also in academic terms. This dominance was exerted via a number of routes, not least through peer pressure, and, if not matched, created a feeling of personal inadequacy and a lower status in the clinical environment. This was compounded by a laudable questioning of 'custom and practice' in which, where criticism was deemed appropriate, individuals, rather than the organisation and its approach to progress, were singled out.

There was a strong desire on the part of the participants to move away from a blame culture to one that recognised failure as an opportunity to learn. A greater tension in this environment had been generated since the introduction of diploma and degree nurse training, in which nurses have been educated to question and challenge practice. This was seen as a positive development, yet the organisations were not always ready to accept that challenge as positive. Instead, it was often perceived as a personal criticism of those who had been practising for many years. There was a clear recognition of a need to move the culture of nursing on, to embrace change and challenge as an opportunity for continuous learning and therefore improved nursing practice and patient care.

It must not, however, be assumed that everything that is custom and usual practice is poor. Many activities undertaken by nurses, while not based on academic research, have been honed over many decades to achieve best practice. There is unquestionably a research element in this approach, based on reflection, that, when ultimately refined, can change care delivery. This is well described by Freshwater (2000) as the continual review and reflection of actions to change practice. These actions have been a natural part of nursing, albeit often unrecognised, and have in the main created nursing as it is today. It must therefore be accepted into practice and encouraged as a fundamental part of the professional nursing culture.

Organisation

The working environment was identified as the next most important aspect of influencing positive and negative learning, the need for reflective practice being stressed. Critical incidents were identified as a useful tool by which to introduce reflective practice, an activity underpinned by the implementation of clinical supervision. Not surprisingly, many of the issues raised in association with good learning are reflected in the discussions on how to progress clinical practice. Box 5.8 makes clear the principles of good learning through formal and informal mechanisms. The environment in which we work was seen to be a major influence on personal and professional expectation. This would clearly be compounded by many intrinsic factors such as local leadership and team values.

Nursing is monopolised by the clinical setting. The relationship between education, academia and practice, with apparently differing values and goals, was seen by the group participants to be distant. There needs to be a more visible merging of values and goals between academia and the NHS in order to facilitate the future development of the nursing profession. This is not a one-way track and the sole responsibility of one or other of the organisations. Skills and competencies are the responsibility of both academic and clinical institutions, being not simply localised but universalised.

Box 5.8
The principles of good learning

Positive

- Reflective practice:
  - **formal**: structured review of a experience
  - **informal**: unconscious review of experience at the end of working day
- Recognised competencies that underpin practice development
- Universally agreed competencies
- Visual impact of facility, either clinical or academic
  - attractive and comprehensive displays and information leaflets
  - accessible policies and protocols that are up to date and relevant

Negative

- Difficult or bad experience not subjected to reflection on the part of the team or the individual
- Learning without identifying expectations and competencies – goals never achieved
- Cluttered surroundings, out-of-date information, old policies and protocols that are not subjected to review or audit

---

There is no mystery to learning and no monopoly of its ownership. It is now the right of every nurse to learn both in the daily clinical routine and within a properly supervised academic environment. The appropriate place to learn must be determined by the learner and by the needs of the organisation. Learning must be seen as an opportunity to achieve change and therefore excellence. Everyone learns in a different way, and at a different pace, so the leaders of education and practice must facilitate this in ensuring accessibility. The concept of continuous professional development is an essential part of daily practice and is stressed in the statutory requirement to maintain a professional portfolio (Hull and Redfern, 1996). Nurse leaders must develop the skills to enable and facilitate the recognition of learning needs in order to meet the working practices of the care process they work within, ensuring relevance to both clinical care and the individual practitioner.

Many of the issues raised under the heading of 'attitudes' focus on leadership qualities as well as the requisites of a receptive workforce. This is a recurrent theme and is discussed in more detail at the end of this chapter.

Box 5.9

Attitudes

Positive

- Supportive leader who facilitates opportunity

- Understanding relationship between tutor and student, creating an opportunity for both parties to learn from the experience

- Ground rules and expectations that are agreed between tutor and student

- Agreement to recognise time allocation for learning

- Identification of learning needs through regular performance review

Negative

- Poor leadership – dismisses need and opportunity

- Being talked at

- No agreement of expectation

- No agreement of time required

Strategy for success: leadership

It is very easy for readers fairly familiar with the NHS to say sagely to themselves, 'well, there is nothing new here, I knew all that!' In this chapter, we have sought to draw out the agreed views of a large group of nurses and midwives who, when given the time to stand back and reflect, have identified feasible ways (rather than blue-skies scenarios) by which to achieve the professional and personal goals that most of us hold dear. There is now, perhaps more than ever before, a culture of strong motivation, a 'free to give it a go' mentality, which, hand in hand with a supportive, blame-free organisation, will encourage motivation and expectations of success. In a culture that is blame free and non-judgemental, a well-educated workforce can achieve enormous empowerment and success.

Professional leadership

The chain that links all the issues discussed throughout this chapter, which is often invisible but always strong, is leadership. There is no template for leadership, and while there are recognised skills and competencies involved, these skills and competencies should more importantly be aligned with the needs of the local population being served and the shared values of those serving. Having a passion for the provision of quality care is not enough, but it goes a long way towards achieving success. By building a sound knowledge base, the passion can strongly influence the organisation in which you work, so that it can support and facilitate you in your aims. Every nurse has the potential to be leader and at times may be one. A recognition of this will strengthen the influence nurses exert during their leadership episode, which may be over a brief period, through a specific activity or for a longer duration over strategic development.

Leadership does not equate with hierarchy, which is a difficult and complex issue for nursing to digest, given its 'below stairs' history and its previous minority status in the circles of power. It is a dynamic process, and the individual has to be knowledgeable and confident in grasping the moment at which they are the best person to take any issue forward. How does the organisation empower people to feel free to take on leadership when appropriate? Leadership has to start at the top – creating a freedom that is accessible only from the board. This can be achieved only by strong articulation from the 'top' down and must be supported by substantive action and at the same time by recognising that, once that control has been given away, the board may not always agree with the decision made by the local end. There must be a recognition, and acceptance, of clinical values that are based on the recognition of clinical expertise rather than the views of managerial 'grey suits'.

For readers this means looking for a working environment indicating clinical structures that are supported and decision-making being taken close to the patient. For example, has the organisation encouraged the development of nurse consultants, and are clinical specialists well established and working with a degree of autonomy? Do the clinical structures reflect the needs of patients and clients rather than the convenience of the organisation? Do they match the clinical needs of the patients being served within that clinical process? Are staff support systems such as clinical supervision in place? When considering working for an organisation, ask these questions as the answers may offer clear indices of the organisational culture and its commitment to supporting clinical staff.

With the justifiable demands of the professional for a supportive and modern organisation comes responsibility; there is so such thing as a free moan. Nurses have been accustomed to the latter because of the restrictive hierarchy in which they have existed, but now, along with the demand for professional recognition, there is a need to face up to accountability. Nurses have often been able to see the need for change, but because of the culture, traditions and social structures within the health service, which have grown over many years, they have not been able to effect it. The NHS has, however, moved on, and nurses now have to be prepared to rise to the challenge, recognising their accountability and their influential position to help to achieve a change agenda. The history of healthcare in the 21st century must record a recognition of the opportunity that nurses took in shaping the health system by understanding and accepting the responsibility of its power base, thus acknowledging (Littlewood, 1989, p. 229):

> having a major impact on the quality of life and in understanding the meanings patients give to their life and their suffering, the nurse is the best placed healthcare professional to negotiate between the goals of the doctor and the goals of the patient.

Geese are quoted as having the ideal model of leadership. The front flier, or leader, may get weary, and when the encouraging honks of the others are insufficient to maintain its strength, it will fall back into the body of the group and be replaced by another, stronger goose. If a goose falls to the ground, sick, others will stay beside it until its recovery or death. There are lessons to be learned from this model. Nurses need not only to look to the organisation to support them, but also to learn to support each other more than is currently the norm, taking the qualities of caring beyond the convenient confines of those who are sick. Leadership is not simply a matter of charisma, or of a big ego having a fling: it is about establishing continuity, about breaking paths and reaching out a strong hand to those around. It is, quite simply, having, albeit temporarily, the ownership of agreed strategies or actions. Successful leadership does this in partnership.

Conclusion

The discussions that arose between 60 nurses and midwives have been presented, within both an anecdotal and a research context. While it can be claimed with justification that nothing new emerged from the discussions, the approach adopted was a very positive one, allowing a reflection and consideration of productive ways forward for each individual and for those in key organisational roles. Advancing clinical practice cannot occur in isolation and cannot be the product of a new way of teaching or of new clinical discoveries. Improved clinical practice can only be generated through a matrix of activities and, most importantly, attitudinal approaches (see Figure 2.7).

A clinician is responsible for providing individual care of high quality and for being able to demonstrate this by setting and monitoring standards of care. Collaborative standard-setting in which more than one clinician is involved must be agreed, central to this collaboration being a shared philosophy of care. There are now formal structures in place to help to assure this, these being discussed in Chapters 2 and 4. Understanding the mechanisms of change and appreciating the value of change are also discussed (see Chapter 1), but none of this is worth the paper it is written on if the individual professional is not committed to excellence. To advance clinical practice is not an irregular activity; it is a state of mind that can only be comfortable for the individual if he or she is empowered and willing to accept the challenge. It is certainly a challenge worth accepting.

Key Point Summary

- Develop a 'have a go' culture

- Make time to question practices

- Value each other and say 'thank you'

- Employ lifelong learning

Suggested further reading

Abbott, P. and Sapsford, R. (eds) (1993) *Research into Practice*. Milton Keynes: Open University Press.

Holloway, I. and Wheeler, S. (1996) *Qualitative Research for Nurses*. Oxford: Blackwell Science.

Mikkelsen, B. (1995) *Methods for Development Work and Research. A Guide for Practitioners*. London: Sage.

Fox, D. (1982) *Fundamentals of Research in Nursing*. Norwalk, CT: Appleton-Century-Crofts.

Bishop, V. (ed.) (1999) *Working Towards a Research Degree. Insights from the Nursing Perspective*. London: NTBooks.

6

Partnerships and Power in Care

Tom Tait and Jeanette Higginson

This chapter seeks systematically to examine the notion of power in nursing and how it can impact upon the relationship between nurse, informal carer and patient. The relationship between the patient, the informal carer and the nurse has come under greater scrutiny as government policies drive a strong agenda of improved consultation and greater consumer involvement in healthcare. This philosophical shift requires nurses to reappraise the roles normally adopted within the care process, as well as to acknowledge that power relationships will need to change to accommodate more equal, patient-focused care interventions. The tension between the nurse's duty of care and the patient's right to self-determination within the care partnership is explored in depth.

Christensen (1993) describes the nurse–patient partnership as an opportunity to look at what happens when a nurse offers expertise to a person in his or her care. This specialised assistance is required to help to minimise the impact upon the person, and the family, of a healthcare problem and its associated treatment regime. To aid the development of a constructive, therapeutic nurse–patient partnership, the importance of considering individual differences cannot be overstated. People's experience of illness or disability will never be the same, and it is also true to say that their ability to participate actively in their healthcare regime depends upon many factors, including their understanding, their informal support network, and the type of relationship they develop with those directly involved in their care.

Abdel-Halim (1983) remarks on the tendency, in nursing, to consider that participation is good – and that means good for everyone. It must be accepted that patient participation in any healthcare programme is not absolute. People's levels of participation will differ, but the major care goal must be to enable people to take control of their health whenever possible. Contemporary healthcare today demands that care is based upon forming productive partnerships between nursing staff and those in their care. The formulation and implementation of a robust nurse–patient or nurse–carer partnership in which the patient or service user's needs are the focus of the care plan can only enhance overall patient care and coping mechanisms during the period of ill health.

Partnerships

There are many different partnerships, so it is important to define what *could* constitute a partnership within the confines of the nurse–patient relationship. A dictionary definition of 'partnership' is 'a contractual relationship in which there is a joint venture with a sharing of profits', and Wade (1995) defines 'partnership' as having a number of meanings. These meanings contain elements such as relationships, reciprocity, sharing equality, friendship and participation. Therefore, within the context of these definitions, a contractual relationship would indicate equality between the parties, and the 'profit' could be interpreted as the health of the patient, a view of partnerships in healthcare that is also supported by Hill (1996).

The White Paper *Working for Patients* (DoH, 1989b), advocated the formulation of strong partnerships that would result in increased efficiency and effectiveness. While this vision of a more patient-focused care regime is an exciting concept for nurses to embrace, questions have arisen on how much these practices can drive current clinical practice within the current levels of demand seen in the NHS. Further issues to be considered are those surrounding power (of the healthcare professional), empowerment (of the patient/client) and culture. What skills are needed for the healthcare professional to facilitate such a relationship? The innate and the learned social skills of both the nurse and the patient will have a major impact on the development and shape of any nurse–patient–informal carer partnerships.

Jewell (1994) has suggested that the terms 'patient involvement', 'patient collaboration' and 'partnership' tend to be used interchangeably, while Brownlea et al. (1980), suggest that there is no real consensus on what participation means. It would therefore seem that the meaning of partnership could become confusing to either party. Participation and partnership, however, do appear to go hand in hand. Bernarde and Mayerson (1978) see this as the inevitable outcome of consumerism, the patient–provider relationship now reflecting greater active patient involvement and self-help. Savage (1990), however, argues that this is a reaction to the medical profession's long-standing control of the patient–health professional relationship. The implication of this change of emphasis is that healthcare should aim primarily to restore a patient's autonomy, cure or a restoration of function being secondary aims.

Encouraging patient autonomy appears to reflect the ethical and moral rights of the individual. Dyer and Blosch (1987) contend that the 'notion of partnership' is a reminder that important personal qualities are involved in the pursuit and maintenance of the highest ethical standards, thus enhancing the patient's 'locus of control' (Rotter, 1966). As nursing accounts for about 80 per cent of the direct care that patients receive, and often involves personal and intimate care activities, nurses are in a unique situation to develop a complex form of relationship with patients. Peplau (1969) states that this will involve a level of intimacy and reciprocity that has been described as a 'professional closeness', but Campbell (1984) counters that this may be difficult to achieve in practice, as it will involve a delicate balance of personal involvement.

Reciprocity in the nurse–patient relationship can contribute to a healing process for both participants, 'healing' here meaning 'making whole' rather than 'curing' (McMahon, 1986). One example of this is quoted by a haemodialysis patient who said, 'although the machine may keep me alive, it is the presence of another human being that makes it bearable' (personal communication).

Dimensions of power

Power conjures up images of coercion and domination, an aspect of every social act, the ability to influence or be influenced by something. Foucault's (1980) work suggests that power is as much a productive force as a limitation. In its limiting form, power produces rules. An acknowledgement of the rules creates an awareness of what is forbidden by the rules; for example, a renal patient dependent upon a form of dialysis should be adhering to a diet that is reduced in potassium because of the kidneys' inability to excrete this waste product. The penalty of non-compliance is high. If the patient does not adhere to the recommended diet, he or she is at risk of having a cardiac arrest. Despite the risks, however, some haemodialysis patients do consume food that is not recommended. This apparently childish behaviour needs to be examined carefully by the nurse and handled just as carefully.

It may be that the approach taken with this patient was inappropriate; disempowerment may have encouraged this 'forbidden behaviour' as the individual's ignorance of the relationship between power and knowledge contributes to the maintenance of power in its limiting form. In your own practice, for example, you may observe people displaying a range of behaviours as they seek to redress a perceived power imbalance. Although the disclosure between what is allowed and what is forbidden produces new knowledge, a shift in the power relationship occurs when the acquired knowledge is shared.

Wheeler and Chin (1991) define power as an awareness of one's own strengths and weaknesses, and a deep respect for self and others, the essence being empowerment. A model of power that can be applied to nursing care was identified by Masterson and Maslin-Prothero (1999), who appraise the notion of power in healthcare systems and its impact upon the nurse–patient relationship, citing Lukes (1974) who propounds a theory of three faces or dimensions of power.

One-dimensional power

This idea refers to Dahl's (1961) suggestion that, in order to ascertain who holds power in any relationship, conflict and the outcome of actual decisions have to be observed in order to identify the group or person who holds power. Within a medical model of care, it would, if the interactions of patients and their physicians were observed, be relatively simple to identify who holds the most power.

Second-level power

This concept, according to Masterson and Maslin-Prothero (1999), was developed by Bachrach and Baratz (1962) and cited in Dearlove and Saunders (1984). The notion of second-level power is based upon the assumption of a covert process that acts by suppressing conflicts before they occur. This type of power involves not only the ability to influence the outcome of decisions, but also the ability to dominate the process so that some issues never arise or some decisions never get made. This maintains the status quo. Bachrach and Baratz (1962) criticise the one-dimensional theory described above, reasoning that if the decision-making process alone is examined, the power involved in preventing issues being raised is not being acknowledged.

In relation to nursing practice, the potential for this type of power dimension should not be ignored. From the patient perspective, it could be seen as being counter-productive to question treatment or complain in any way: 'I can't afford to have to wait for a second opinion' or 'why complain, I don't have time to fill in such a lengthy form'. As a practitioner, you need to be aware that the healthcare system in which you work may have hidden but very powerful barriers ensuring that awkward questions are never raised. Supporting, even tacitly, these barriers can only diminish the ability to develop excellence in practice.

Three-dimensional power

Masterson and Maslin-Prothero (1999) state that this type of power is not seen as commonly in individuals or groups but instead shows itself in what Dearlove and Saunders (1984) describe as 'systems of domination'. They suggest that, within systems of dominance, power relationships influence the very structures of society itself and that people's preferences are shaped to such a degree that neither overt nor covert conflict exists. This presupposes that, in such circumstances, power relationships have become so customised that they involve a set of social relationships in which one party has established habitual command over another, such that he or she is rarely challenged.

Masterson and Maslin-Prothero (1999) develop this theory to suggest that rules with an unequal outcome are obeyed as a matter of course without conflict; power is accepted as a normal component of relationships that exist between certain groups in different social settings. This analysis confirms the concept of institutionalised inequality that is underpinned by ideologies such as sexism or racism. It is here that the rules and practices of the institution generate an unequal outcome, regardless of the motives of those who practise them. To put it succinctly, in these circumstances it is the system rather than the individual's behaviour that is biased. In the case of racism, it may not be a case of institutional racism but one of institutional ignorance. In practice, therefore, you could perpetuate an unequal power system with good intent but remain ignorant of how it can impact upon minority groups.

Power, gender and race

Gender

Healthcare professionals work in an increasingly complex multicultural environment in which there is an increased need for a deeper understanding of its constituent groups if 'partnership' is to become the forefront of care delivery. A patient's cultural background and gender will present the nurse with many challenges.

Webb (1986) identified within her research studies with women patients and female nurses that women wanted and needed nurses to give them detailed information about how their bodies work. They wanted to know how they could expect the prescribed care to affect their physical and emotional health, their family and their working life. The perspective that Webb (1986) propounds has a core belief that women want to have greater control over their own lives and health, and that they therefore need information about how their bodies work, the causes of ill health and the advantages and disadvantages of the treatment available. Ashley (1980) believed that women often risk their health by going to male professionals whose working model emphasises rationality, a lack of emotion and obedience to a father figure represented by the male doctor.

Nurses have in the past often acted as advocates for doctors, but Ashley strongly expressed the wish that nurses can become advocates of women, explaining treatment risks and standing by them to promote a community of shared caring. If this wish is to be realised, Webb (1986) suggests that health workers will need to share their knowledge and power, working together in a non-hierarchical way both with patients and among themselves.

Race

Blackman (2000) argues that racial identity is not a stereotype, instead representing a significant aspect of social identity that can be usefully considered independently of other aspects of personality. Black and white racial identity may also be viewed, in a general sense, arising from sub-dominant/oppressed and dominant/oppressor social roles. Similar states can be recognised in identity differentiation between male and female or disabled and able-bodied.

Sir William Macpherson (1999, p. 209) describes institutional racism as:

> that which can be seen or detected in processes, attitudes and behaviour which amount to discrimination through unwitting prejudice, ignorance, thoughtlessness and racist stereotyping which disadvantage minority ethnic people.

It is important for the practitioner to understand and accept that race is a complex concept and that racial identity is not a stereotype. Discussions surrounding race usually focus upon brown-skinned people, the racial identities of white people rarely being considered, yet white nurses will constantly make decisions that can profoundly affect the lives of black people in their care. Similarly, male nurses may make decisions, with good intent, that can impact negatively upon a female patient's well-being.

The question of racial identity has significant implications for healthcare practitioners, and its importance should be reflected in the training and education of healthcare professionals. Racial identities operate at deep, personal, conscious and unconscious levels and significantly influence decision-making. Understanding this is equally important for both black and white healthcare professionals, Blackman (2000) suggesting that, even with the best will in the world, a person's racial identity will influence decision-making and could be instrumental in developing a partnership in which one party will be oppressed. *The nursing care you plan and deliver must therefore be couched in an arena of equal opportunity and anti-racist care that acknowledges cultural differences.* This will require all nurses to understand and learn how to abandon conscious and unconscious racist attitudes.

It is our view that, within the field of learning disability nursing, the current services available within the UK to people with learning disabilities from black and minority ethnic communities have developed through a process moulded by this country's history and social policy (Tait, 1999). The history is fundamentally a white one, and the social policies have evolved to meet the needs of white people generally. What constitute good care practices for people with learning disabilities, such as the 'normalisation principle' and 'community care', are grounded in a set of 'white Western' values. The development of these initiatives does not fully take into account the differing values and circumstances of the rich diversity of people and the different cultures in today's society within the UK.

The implementation of these principles that embody current public policies – those of normalisation and care within the community – has involved a major assumption about society's norms and values. It might, for example, be the norm in the UK for the older adult with learning disability to live in residential care, but this might not currently hold true for someone from the Asian community. This dichotomy was acknowledged in the White Paper *Caring for People* (DoH, 1989c, p. 10) which stated:

> The Government recognises that people from different cultural backgrounds may have particular care needs and problems. Minority communities may have different concepts of community care and it is important that service providers are sensitive to these variations.

Good community care will take account of the circumstances of minority communities and will be planned in consultation with them.

This statement unfortunately is not reflected in the legislation, so there is no statutory requirement for service providers to ensure that services are culturally sensitive.

Within the context of partnership, it must be remembered that all black people in this country experience some disadvantage in most aspects of their lives as a direct result of their colour. Black people are more likely to be victims of crime (Carr-Hill and Drew, 1988), have a higher level of adverse life events (MacCarthy and Craissati, 1989), have poorer general health (Fenton, 1989) and live in poorer-quality housing (Luthera, 1988). Any care partnership that seeks to place the patient or service user at the centre of the care process will need to acknowledge that treating everyone the same does not equate with equality as it does not take into account the patient's special needs. As a healthcare professional, you will need to recognise that people from different cultural groups will often be disadvantaged and unempowered. Consequently, they will require comprehensive and sensitive support in order to access mainstream services and help to restore them to optimum health.

In displaying a willingness to learn and understand traditions and customs other than their own, health professionals have the opportunity to enrich their own lives, enhance their nursing practice and dispel latent prejudices. By equipping yourself with a deeper understanding of the components that constitute institutional racism, and by being sensitive to the issues that oppress people from minority groups, you can begin to plan care in truly equal partnerships with the people in your care.

Power and informal carers

Social, psychological and physical elements are recognised as pivotal dimensions in the structure of human services, and professionals will need to be aware of the types of structure and the underpinning values that drive them. Hughson and Brown (1988) offer some examples of beliefs that are recognised as being fundamental to the practice of professionals in relation to consumers in human services:

- self-determination
- the protection of civil and human rights
- individualisation
- an acknowledgment of humanity.

These beliefs represent a dramatic shift from the care model of previous decades that was driven by predominant values including protection from and of society.

Summerton (2000) questions how paid healthcarers interact with informal carers and considers whether nurse training prepares nurses to perform competently in a partnership that views the relationship between formal and informal carers as equal. Twigg and Atkin (1994) suggest that health professionals perceive carers in one of three ways:

- carer as a resource
- carer as a co-client
- carer as a co-worker.

Within these different perceptions of how the professional may view the informal carer there exists a potential for an unequal relationship. The skills of the informal carer may be seen as merely supporting the professional's care or as in need of the professional's help in some way. The needs of the informal carer may well be viewed as secondary to the needs of the patient.

Taylor (1996) offers a detailed analysis of the tensions that exist in the nurse's role when allowing parental participation in aspects of nursing that the nurse perceives to be technical. The DoH (1991b) offers guidance to healthcare professionals on parental involvement and suggests that parents should be helped to undertake many unfamiliar tasks. Furthermore, parents should, when appropriate, be encouraged to learn any practical procedures that will enable them to care for their child at home after discharge.

Taylor (1996) poses the question of who decides on the appropriateness of parental involvement, and cites the study by Darbyshire (1994) identifying that, while nurses expected parental participation in 'basic mothering', parents at times felt under pressure to participate in care and to establish themselves as 'good parents', feeling observed and criticised. What this suggests is that the move towards a more enabling relationship will require improved communication between those involved in daily care activities and greater flexibility in the nurse–informal carer relationship. Taylor (1996) concludes that if parents are to become true partners in the care of their child, there is a need for open lines of communication. Furthermore, it is argued that, by encouraging parental involvement in care, there has been a transfer of part of the economic costs of caring from the state to the family (Anderson and Elfert, 1989).

Against the backdrop of the 'named nurse' initiative (Dooley, 1999), which stemmed from the Thatcher reforms of the NHS (Read, 1991) and the mandate that every patient should have a named, qualified, nurse, health visitor or midwife, an ideal opportunity exists for nurses to develop a therapeutic relationship with informal carers and patients. Such relationships should allow a significant appreciation of their specific nursing requirements and facilitate the empowerment of the individuals involved. Taylor (1996), for example, offers the hope that, when relationships develop, informal carers may be enabled to discuss their role and negotiate fully in the care of the child. If informal carers are to become more involved in the care process and be seen as a valuable asset within the care team, an enabling, empowering relationship needs to be developed. This requires flexibility on the part of the nurse as informal carer needs are not static, and this flexibility can only be achieved successfully through confidence in one's knowledge base, and through good peer support, such as clinical supervision.

Empowerment

Empowerment is a positive concept in which power is both taken and given (Gibson, 1991). It is a process of helping individuals to develop a critical awareness of the root causes of their problems, as well as a readiness to act upon this awareness. Empowerment is associated with such concepts as mutual support, community organisation, self-esteem and connectedness. Sadly, empowerment is more easily understood through its absence, which is characterised by powerlessness, helplessness, alienation, victimisation, subordination and oppression. Gibbs (1991) argues that these words are all too frequently used by nurses to describe their position in the healthcare arena. O'Donnell (1993) suggests that one may feel threatened by any perceived loss of power. This perceived threat, or loss, can be overcome by a commitment and willingness to empower those in one's care with information and a greater involvement in decision-making.

It would, however, be naive to make the assumption that all people wish to become more knowledgeable about and more involved in their care (Biley, 1992). Some patients may wish to remain ignorant, preferring a parent–child relationship with the nurse. Abdellah and Levine (1957) found that although patients appreciated being involved in the planning of their care, they also wished to be treated with 'firmness'. It has to be recognised that it may not always be possible to achieve a partnership (Teasdale, 1987). Some patients may not be well enough, some may not be capable of making an informed choice, and some may simply not wish to enter into a partnership. Patients may be reluctant collaborators and opt for defining the 'rules' so that they can behave in the manner they perceive to be expected of them (Waterworth and Luker, 1990).

This suggests that some patients feel forced into taking a share of the control of their care, and in some cases this may be so, but current government policy to make partnerships in healthcare is based on the reality of a public that, with improved education and concomitantly higher expectations, seeks to be informed and involved in any decisions relating to its healthcare (Kawik, 1995). The onus is therefore upon practitioners to ensure that these concepts underpin their professional practice.

Care partnerships

The 'partnership' approach has been cited by the DoH (1989b, 1991b) and the Audit Commission (1993) as being the way forward, yet there are currently too few studies on nursing that evaluate the benefits of this approach upon the care processes. There is, however, some evidence to suggest that active patient participation leads to an improved outcome and better patient adjustment (Wilson-Barnett and Fordham, 1982). Similarly, it has been demonstrated that there is a difference in the way in which nurses and patients perceive care (Jacobs, 1980; Smith et al., 1980).

Interest in the area of patient/informal carer involvement in decision-making is increasing. This collaborative approach requires the nurse to empower patients and their informal carers to work as equal partners by sharing knowledge, values, responsibility, outcomes and visions (Henneman et al., 1995). In order for these concepts to be fully incorporated into practice, it may be necessary for nurses to examine their own values and belief systems. Here continuing professional development plays an important role by encouraging practitioners to explore their practice in areas such as family dynamics, role clarification, negotiation, communication skills and reflection.

If you develop a relationship that is therapeutic and trusting, this benefits not only the patient, but also the practitioner, through increased role satisfaction. This type of relationship demands honesty, with open lines of communication, discussions on possible care strategies, being straightforward and talking in a language that all can understand. Contemporary nursing practice demands greater patient involvement in care. Some nurses may still feel threatened with this approach as it requires the nurse to practise within an arena of greater autonomy. By entering into a democratic relationship that views the patient/informal carer as an equal, valued partner, the patient or informal carer will have increased feelings of self-worth. This enhanced esteem will help to create a platform on which improved consultations and negotiations will form the basis of a care plan that is 'owned', valued and understood by all partners.

Within a care partnership, four key roles have been identified that the nurse fulfils:

- carer
- supporter
- teacher
- referrer to other disciplines.

This partnership model, first propounded by Casey (1988), lends itself to identifying significant nursing functions in the hope of establishing a relationship of equality between professional carers and the parents of children in receipt of nursing care. Although this model makes a distinction between informal or family care and nursing care activities, it does not advocate fixed boundaries and can therefore be applied within other nursing fields.

In this context, the nurse as a carer should perform nursing procedures or give skilled care only when appropriate. That is, the nurse will only become involved if the patient or family members do not have the appropriate skills or knowledge to ensure a successful healthcare outcome. As a supporter, the nurse must implement strategies that enable significant family members or the patient to become involved in caregiving. This demonstrates a sense of trust between all parties. Such a relationship is essential if patients are to perceive that they are partners in care and indeed have a valuable contribution to make. A stated objective of the 'partnership in care' model is to enable the patient and family members to meet healthcare needs with minimal intervention from healthcare professionals.

Some problems will, however, require specialist skills and knowledge. To achieve a policy of minimal intervention, the nurse must assess family knowledge, skills and attitudes, and devise a suitable teaching programme that enhances knowledge and understanding. While this partnership model acknowledges that nursing care is unique, it also recognises that nurses may need to refer to other disciplines in pursuit of achieving the care goals. This multi-disciplinary approach ensures that maximum family support is maintained.

An example of this multi-dimensional role in practice can be illustrated by that of the community renal nurse, or continuous ambulatory peritoneal dialysis nurse, whose sole responsibility is that of carer, supporter, teacher and, if necessary, referrer. Casey's (1988) model clearly identifies within an ethos of shared responsibility what the nurse's role is and how the nurse is expected to function within the parameters of the partnership. The challenge for the nurse is to put into practice what has for so long been a fundamental belief across the profession – that patients are their own most appropriate carers, both in health and in sickness. It is, however, important to remember that a strong commitment to this approach must not unwittingly compel all patients and informal carers to participate in their care. People should be allowed to define the level of involvement with which they are most comfortable. Any pressure from the nurse that requires other parties to undertake an increased technical role could be counter-productive if they have neither the skills nor the confidence to fulfil that role.

A partnership approach provides a valuable medium for assessing, planning, implementing and evaluating nursing care, focusing upon the patients' perception of need and their role within the care processes. A number of practical strategies have helped to facilitate improved nurse–patient partnerships, the most notable of which is primary nursing. In this, the underpinning philosophy (Pontin, 1999) creates the conditions for an empowering relationship between all partners that will help to maintain the stability and integrity of the family unit during a time of adverse family stress.

Elliott and Turrell (1996) explore the nurse's role within the nurse–patient–informal carer partnership and cite Saunders (1995), who cautions that some may feel that the nurse's role has been eroded as more emphasis is placed upon patient participation and self-care. Malin and Teasdale (1991) suggest that nurses adopt a caring role when they do things for patients, or when they protect them from harm or necessary worry, and that nurses adopt an empowering role when they put their skills and knowledge at the disposal of the patient, whom they trust to make responsible decisions.

It can be seen from these illustrations that tension will exist between the different roles that nurses may adopt in seeking to develop a therapeutic relationship with those in their care. What is clear in a patient-focused healthcare environment is that nurses will have to re-evaluate their roles, motives and skills, realigning them, as Elliott and Turrell (1996) suggest, to counter any traditional practices that have, perhaps unwittingly, given them power over patients by giving priority to professional need.

Malin and Teasdale (1991) propound that the empowering role of nurses will require them to place their clinical expertise at the disposal of those in their care rather than assuming that the patient automatically affirms clinical opinion. Elliott and Turrell (1996) further suggest that theoretically, in this context, the nurse has a responsibility to care or treat only if patients wish to avail themselves of the nursing skills on offer, a view that may appear contentious, as it is presumed that, when people enter healthcare institutions, they wish to receive such care and expertise.

The UKCC (1992b) *Code of Professional Conduct* requires the nurse to act to protect the safety of the patient rather than in a way that will undermine their condition and interests. This can prove to be problematic when respecting patients' wishes. A renal patient, for example, who has a low haemoglobin level may refuse a blood transfusion for religious reasons. The nurse could adopt a strategy of negotiation with the patient and explore possible courses of action that may achieve the desired health gain outcome. But it is the patient who will ultimately decide what healthcare is 'best' for him or her. Nurses' perception of their duty to care could, in this case, cause conflict and dissonance.

A situation may arise when a patient, by virtue of their intellectual capacity, may not be able to enter into the nurse's notion of a collaborative partnership. Baldwin (1999) argues that all too often practitioners will over-ride decisions made by a person with a learning disability in the belief that it is the wrong choice. Dix and Gilbert (1995) suggest that the assumption by the professional that they are better able than the person in their care to know what is, or is not, in the patient's best interests could be an expression of paternalism. A decision made by a person with a learning disability may be perceived as wrong simply because it was not the choice the professional would have made.

While autonomy and paternalism are part of our everyday life, they become an issue when we fall ill. Jones (1996) cites the work of Dworkin (1988), who suggests that there are many definitions of 'autonomy' and cautions against the assumption that different theorists are all alluding to the same thing when they use this term. Dworkin does, however, identify two features common to all definitions: that autonomy relates to persons, and that it is a desirable quality. Tschudin (1989) points out that individuals, however freethinking, are still social beings. This means that we are influenced by social factors and that the concept of autonomy must therefore be seen as relative.

Melia (1989) defined paternalism as healthcare professionals making choices about the treatment of clients that they deemed to be in those clients' 'best interests'. It is suggested that this may be an uncomfortable issue to confront, possibly because it challenges us to question what nursing really means and to appraise our motives for entering a caring profession. Jones (1996) offers the example of the conflict arising between the patient's right to autonomy and the practitioner's duty of care when a person for whom we are caring makes an autonomous decision that will result in some self-harm. The dichotomy is often resolved by the use (consciously or unconsciously) of paternalistic action by nursing and medical staff.

Rumbold (1986) draws attention to the vulnerability of patients. Illness can cause people to become confused, weak or anxious. If this state inhibits a person's ability to self-advocate, autonomy is seriously affected. This vulnerability could be increased if staff attitudes towards patients were such that assumptions were made on their behalf. Such beliefs may include rationalisations by nurses that 'ignorance is bliss' or 'people are incapable of understanding'. Jones (1996) suggests that doctors must consider their patients' opinions when deciding what course of action to take.

It has been observed that nurses who practise from a paternalistic stance view their colleagues who practise from a model of autonomy as uncaring or disinterested, while those practising from an autonomy model may view their paternalistic colleagues as bombastic and inflexible.

Empowerment and risk-taking

Carson (1995) identifies that the concept of risk is by nature complex, and its assessment will be both subjective and situation dependent. Perske (1972) suggests that risk is necessary for normal human development and that carers, by being over-zealous in protecting the individual from possible harm, can deny them valuable experiences and opportunities. Heyman and Huckle (1993) demonstrated how carers, both formal and informal, can be disabling and indeed further disable people with learning disabilities by limiting their competencies and by hampering their development of social relationships.

Baldwin (1999) concludes that the issue of risk is one that requires careful attention from those providing services for people with learning disabilities. It is important that risks are assessed and managed in ways that, while protecting both patient and public from harm, still allow for individual growth and development. This approach will mean giving the opportunity and power to make a decision that may involve some degree of risk. Within the other branches of nursing, this analysis of risk can be applied to many situations in which patients and formal and informal carers debate issues surrounding treatment. Within the parameters of an individual's right to self-determination and a nurse's duty of care provision, the potential exists for a care strategy to be agreed acknowledging both concepts while ensuring that the power base is shared equally between all parties.

Summary

There is clearly no single approach that will encompass all the issues raised in this chapter. Working in partnership is a broad dimension that is context dependent and subject to one's personal beliefs and professional values. Equality, racial sensitivity, enabling, valuing, empowering, trusting and self-determining are all prerequisites for a therapeutic partnership between care professionals, the patient and the family. As a nurse, you will need to acknowledge the tensions that exist within your relationships with people within your sphere of responsibility, as well as to explore strategies to facilitate more dynamic and robust care partnerships that place patients and their families at the centre of the care process and support you in meeting these challenges.

You will also need to develop democratic and sensitive ways of working with a range of professional colleagues. Such partnerships should affirm the individual's intrinsic worth and the unique contribution that they can make to their own healthcare. A partnership that accepts individual differences and constantly seeks to empower all participants to make a meaningful and valuable contribution to the nursing care plan is truly therapeutic.

Key Point Summary

- The patient/carer relationship needs to be democratic
- All members of the healthcare team have a power basis
- Gender and race will have an impact on care processes
- Care partnerships need to be nurtured
- There will always be tensions between autonomy and paternalism

7

Informatics and IT in Nursing Practice

Denis Anthony

Clinical nurses are finding information technology (IT) increasingly useful. Some of the more common IT facilities are:

- *hospital information support systems (HISSs)*
- *databases*
- *online resources of an increasing diversity available on the NHS intranet (NHSNet), via Trusts' own intranets or from the Internet itself.*

Nurses in the clinical area should not bother about the technology itself but instead consider what it might offer to them in their practice. Typical nursing functions that are helped by IT include:

- *evidence-based practice and research: using bibliographic databases (especially where a full text of the articles or abstracts is available), full text electronic journals and online clinical guidelines*
- *continuing professional development: using online courses, online continuing education articles and electronic discussion forums*
- *planning and executing nursing care: sharing electronic patient records with other health professionals and accessing HISSs*
- *patient information: either writing new material or using material made available from other Trusts/organisations.*

This chapter will explore the use of IT in nursing practice, concentrating on those aspects of IT which assist the nurse practically. We will start with an outline of some of the more important

concepts and resources, much of which may already be familiar.
This material is not covered here in depth but it is available in
many texts, for example Anthony (1996).

This chapter contains many components, and you may wish to
look at only one or a few to start with. My experience is that
readers are only interested in IT when it helps them to do their
clinical job. You might want, for example, to provide patient
information on the Internet, so you would go to the end of the
chapter and ignore all the information on clinical guidelines and
so on, which is not immediately useful to you.

The important thing to bear in mind when reading this chapter
is that it is not important to learn about computing. You will
want to use technology to obtain information on your patients,
or to provide information for your patients, or to assist you in
your studies so that you can improve your care of patients, or to
help your students by providing coursework. In all cases, it is
patient care that is the central purpose, either directly in the
clinical situation or indirectly by education and improving your
nursing skills.

If at any time while reading this chapter you feel inadequate
with respect to your IT or computing skills, I have failed. You
do not need to be a computing specialist to use IT systems, any
more than you need to be a mechanic to drive your car, or be
a plumber to take a bath. Many nurses and other health workers
are questioning the use of the term 'information technology',
preferring 'informatics'. This new term stresses the use of information, which need not be based on computers at all. Informatics
looks at paper information systems or information generated
during conversations (ward hand-overs, for example) as well as
computer systems. I have, however, kept to the older and more
restricted term as most people are more familiar with this term,
and almost all the information I am considering in this chapter
can best be dealt with using computers and computer networks.

While you can use information without computers, I suggest
that, in the 21st century, this will restrict you. Traditional paper-
based information is still highly relevant and useful, and you
will continue to use professional journals and books, as indeed
I do. Informal and formal conversations with colleagues and
patients are vital and will still be used. IT is not meant to be a

replacement for these other excellent systems, but it can produce powerful systems with the ability to access information in ways that were previously impossible.

If you are in a remote area, for example, and you have a clinical emergency, it is very useful to speak to a specialist using old technology (the telephone), but new technology employing video cameras attached to a computer network allows the specialist to view the patient from a computer terminal possibly hundreds of miles away. More down to earth uses are emerging for this form of communication. Elderly frail people can have video surveillance in their homes, connected to a central site where carers can keep an eye on the residents.

As a further example, consider the ward sister in a small cottage hospital. She has 16 beds and is the most senior member of staff. She is 16 miles from the nearest library in Leicester. The tissue viability nurse for the Trust is on maternity leave, and a temporary replacement has yet to be appointed. This is a problem as the ward sister wants to know how best to debride sloughy leg ulcers, common among her patients. She accesses the Internet from a computer attached via a modem in her office (this is increasingly realistic as computers and modems are cheap, and simply use the telephone line, charged at the local call rate). She searches through Medline (available free on the Internet from many sources) and locates several evidence-based articles on debridement, but fails to locate a systematic review. The information informs her clinical practice and suggests an area for a future review. The sister contacts by electronic mail (email) the NHS Centre for Reviews and Dissemination (CRD) and asks whether a review does exist, and if not, whether they could consider this.

The above examples illustrate some of the capabilities of IT in clinical situations. The rest of the chapter will explore a few more but does not attempt to cover all areas.

Computer concepts

Personal computers and word processing

Only a few years ago most nurses had not used a personal computer (PC) or a word processor (WP). Today most of us use a PC every day, the single most common use for one being to write documents using a WP. I am not going to discuss PCs or WPs here as they are so commonplace. However, WPs, typified by Microsoft Word, allow you to create documents more efficiently and effectively.

Local area networks

While many nurses access the Internet from home using a PC attached to a modem using the telephone system, at work they are more likely to be using a local area network (LAN). A LAN is a network of computers in the near vicinity to each other; it could, for example, link the computers in one hospital site. LANs allow users to share information, send email across the LAN, access patient records and so on. Thus they allow a local group of users to communicate and share information.

Electronic patient record

In a multi-disciplinary health service, keeping separate records in different locations, and having medical, nursing and professions allied to medicine all keeping their own notes, can cause confusion. A unified record held electronically has obvious advantages (and some problems, in for example the security of the record). To professionals' records we can add laboratory reports and other data on the patient. Such systems are already in place, typically utilising commercial HISSs (see below). The main advantage of the unified record is that the data are always available and are accessible by all the team, to whom legitimate access has been granted. This can only be achieved using an electronic system.

Tele-medicine

This is medicine at a distance, using electronic means. An example might be use of video camera attached to a network to allow a physician to see a patient and give a diagnosis.

The Internet, intranets and NHSNet

The Internet is a giant worldwide network of computers. When you access the Internet, you have potential access to any other computer attached to the Internet (although you may not in practice be allowed to access some of them). This allows organisations and individuals to place on line information for public use. Thus commercial companies can use the Internet to advertise their services, and users can order goods and so on via the Internet. Universities can place information about courses, charities outline their target area, and governments place White Papers and other public documents on line.

Nurses are increasingly accessing the Internet for professional development, either from home, using an Internet Provider (IP), or at work (in many cases using NHSNet; see below). Users typically access information using a program called a browser, such as Netscape or Internet Explorer. A massive increase in interest has recently occurred in the Internet, specifically the World Wide Web (WWW; see below), which is but one (albeit very important) facility that you can use on the Internet. The Internet can be accessed via your PC or from a LAN.

Many organisations have what is called an intranet. This is essentially an Internet system that is available to a restricted group of people; one example of an intranet is the NHS's NHSNet. This uses methods of transferring information similar to those of the Internet, and it has similar resources such as Web browsers to access information, but it is accessible only to authorised NHS staff. Information that is sensitive may be placed on an intranet, but information for public access is best placed on the Internet. Many Trusts have their own intranet, on which material that is intended only for NHS staff is put. This is often not strictly sensitive data but may include Trust documentation, training and so on, material that is of little interest outside the Trust. The Trust will typically also have an Internet site to allow patients or potential patients to access information that will be useful to help them prepare for surgery, for example.

As an example of networked computers, consider the situation of the Glenfield Hospital and Leicester Royal Infirmary Trusts, both in Leicester. Both of these hospitals have intranets, and in both cases there is a WWW-based information system on the intranet. Thus users of the Internet have to learn no new system as they will be familiar with the WWW. In the Leicester Royal Infirmary, local groups are allowed to have their information placed on the intranet, where details of nursing research projects undertaken locally in the Trust are summarised. Glenfield Trust has a system whereby local authorised users may upload the information directly onto the intranet. Staff in such a system 'own' their data. The technical staff manage the site and produce systems to allow the users to upload the data without needing any technical skills.

The World Wide Web

The WWW is a hypertext system, meaning that its documents contain links to other documents, which may be accessed directly from the first one. Links can also be made to pictures, video, sound and so on. These linked documents may be located on the same computer as the document from which they are linked, but this is not necessary. The linked document can be anywhere on the Internet; it could even be located on a different continent. This makes for a very powerful information system. You can create WWW pages of local guidelines (for example, for pressure sores) and link these to a review of the treatment of pressure sores at the NHS CRD, as well as to the US-based National Guideline Clearinghouse, which has several guidelines for pressure sores.

Figure 7.1 is an example of a WWW page (taken from an article in *Nursing Standard Online*). In this case, it is devoted to clinical guidelines, and there are links (underlined) that, in most browsers, are identified by a different colour. If you click on this link, you are taken directly to the linked document, in this case the US National Guideline Clearinghouse, which has many clinical guidelines (Figure 7.2). Entering 'diabetic foot' as a search item located the item in Figure 7.3.

So we were able to locate, from the pages of a UK nursing journal, a US site with clinical guidelines, and having accessed the latter (simply by clicking on a link), we were able to search it for the item of interest to us (in this case the diabetic foot). Finally, we came up with a clinical guideline.

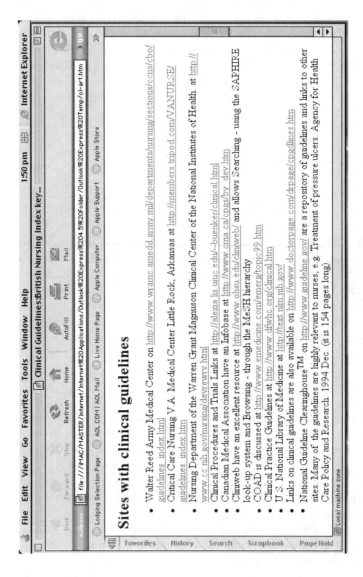

Figure 7.1 Example of a World Wide Web page

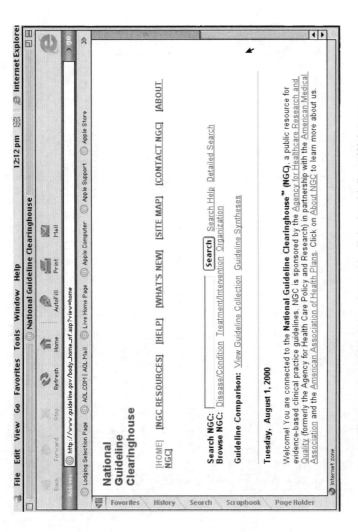

Figure 7.2 Link from sites with clinical guidelines Web page

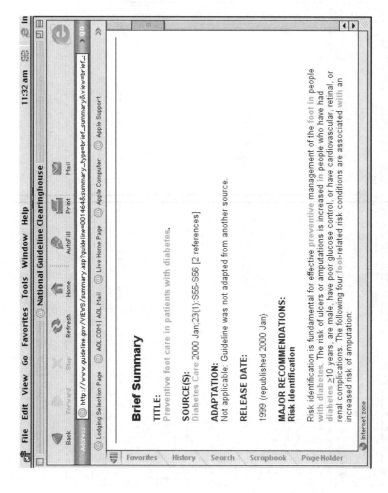

Figure 7.3 Link from National Guideline Clearinghouse Web page

Email and email lists

One of the major uses of computer networks is to allow individual users to communicate with each other. One method of doing this is email, whereby messages are sent from one individual to another. Email can be sent over a local network (for example, a Trust LAN) or over the Internet (or another large network).

Email lists are communities of email users with a common interest. If one member sends a message to the list (which has its own special email address), all the members receive the email message. Email lists can be organisational – all nurses in a Trust or all members of a university faculty for example; such lists are 'closed' to people outside the organisational group. Most email lists are formed around a subject, for example nursing in the UK or diabetes, these lists typically being open to anyone who wants to join them.

Uniform resource locators

To locate information on the WWW and other Internet resources, you need to know its address, which is called the uniform resource locator (URL). The URL can be typed in on your Web browser, if you are online, to access the resource, which could be an online journal, a government report or the personal home page of a student nurse or a charity. Databases such as Medline can also be accessed via the WWW. URLs are typically of the form http://<address>, for example http://www.dmu.ac.uk is the URL of my university. With most WWW browsers, you can dispense with the first bit (http://); thus typing www.dmu.ac.uk as an address in your browser will in most cases get you De Montfort University home page.

Databases

Online bibliographic databases can be accessed to address specific clinical queries and to provide evidence-based care. In the clinical area, nurses may also have access to specialised databases, for example to look up poisons in the case of an overdose.

Some of the most relevant online bibliographic databases to nursing include the Bath Information Data Services, Medline, CINAHL and the English National Board for Nursing, Midwifery and Health Visiting database. These allow health workers to identify articles and in some cases access the abstract or even the full text of an article.

Online journals

Many journals are available on the Internet, including the full text of the whole journal (which may only be available on the Internet, that is, a purely electronic journal, or it may be a mirror of a paper copy), a partial online copy of a paper journal (for example *Nursing Standard*, which has about half its copy available online) or simply 'webverts', in which information about a journal is given.

Subject directories

There is so much on the Internet that you are unlikely to know the most relevant sites for your purpose. There are methods of searching the Internet using built-in search 'engines' on most browsers, but the results can be very unfocused and many of the returned sites are irrelevant. A search for sites using the keyword 'nurse', for example, gave information on sharks (nurse sharks), babies (nursing mothers) and pornography!

For specialised subjects, you may be better off accessing an online directory. These are maintained by specialists and consist of a list of sites, known to be useful in the given subject, which is regularly updated. For UK nurses, the best such list – Nursing and Healthcare Resources on the Internet – is currently based at the University of Sheffield and run by a lecturer in nursing, Rod Ward; it is at http://www.shef.ac.uk/~nhcon.

Government papers concerning IT and information in health

The NHS and the government have published many reports, both Green and White Papers. Recent reports that are relevant to nursing practice include the following:

Reviewing Health Information Services: ETD Support for LIS Development (NHS Information Authority, 1999a).
Information for Health: An Information Strategy for the Modern NHS 1998–2005. A National Strategy for Local Implementation (DoH, 1998a).
The New NHS: Modern, Dependable: A National Framework for Assessing Performance (DoH, 1998b).
A First Class Service: Quality in the New NHS (DoH, 1998, 1998a, b, 1999; NHS Information Authority, 1999a, b; NHSE, 1994a, b, c, 1995, 1996b, 1997a).

All of the above are available online from the UK government Web site (http://www.open.gov), and/or the DoH Web site (http://www.doh.gov.uk/); *A First Class Service: Quality in the New NHS*, for example, is at http://www.doh.gov.uk/newnhs/quality.htm.

The remainder of this chapter concentrates on how the above help you, the practising nurse, to do your job, specifically on how the Internet, intranets, LANs and the resources available on these networks help nurses practically. This chapter does *not* attempt to cover the curriculum for nursing informatics as suggested by the Enabling People project (http://www. enablingpp.exec.nhs.uk), as this would need a complete book.[1]

Neither does it attempt to discuss all the clinical systems that a nurse might find, as these vary from Trust to Trust. Instead, I shall attempt to give a flavour of what IT can offer the clinical nurse to assist *practically*. I shall concentrate on WWW services on the Internet. This is not as large a restriction as it might appear, as NHSNet applications will typically use similar interfaces, and Trusts are increasingly using both the Internet and Internet-like intranets to distribute information. There is no reason why clinical systems cannot use Web-based products, and online courses will tend also to use a Web-based tutorial product.

With the current demand for clinical governance, I have given a higher proportion of the space of this chapter to clinical guidelines as an example of one of the most important aspects of governance, as well as substantial sections on other evidence-based material.

Each section has a resources list associated with it so you can explore further. Short case studies, which are unashamedly based on my own experience in the East and West Midlands, are presented as examples. I have also provided exercises for reflection.

Clinical governance

Clinical governance is a concept that the Government White Paper *A First Class Service: Quality in the New NHS* recommended to the NHS:

> Clinical governance will be the process by which each part of the NHS quality-assures its clinical decisions. Backed by a new statutory duty of quality, clinical governance will introduce a system of continuous improvement into the NHS. (DoH, 1998a)

The DoH has issued several documents that support clinical governance and clinical guidelines (DoH, 1998a, 1999c; Mann, 1996; NHSE, 1996a, 1997b, 1998a, b, c).

At a national level, clinical guidelines are being addressed by the NICE, whose role will be to assess treatment regimes. It has already given guidance on specific drugs and will be issuing guidelines on a wide range of common clinical problems, including diabetes, heart disease, depression, schizophrenia and pressure sores, to ensure cost-effectiveness as well as clinical effectiveness.

Resource list

Some useful URLs for exploring clinical governance are:

- *A First Class Service: Quality in the New NHS:* http://www.doh.gov.uk/newnhs/quality.htm and a summary at http://www.doh.gov.uk/newnhs/qualsum.htm

- an explanation of clinical governance for primary care group constituents: http://www.doh.gov.uk/ntro/queiss.htm
- a primary care clinical governance page: http://www.doh.gov.uk/pricare/clingov.htm
- *Clinical Governance: Quality in the New NHS:* http://www.doh.gov.uk/pub/docs/doh/hsc065.pdf giving detailed advice on how to implement clinical governance
- local initiatives, which cover a range of approaches to clinical governance, on http://www.doh.gov.uk/nyro/clingov/initia.htm

Organisations

Several organisations have specific information on clinical governance:

- The University of Leicester has a Clinical Governance Research and Development Unit on http://www.le.ac.uk/genpractice/gpaudit/
- A summary of guidelines on clinical governance produced by the Royal College of General Practitioners in association with the NHS Alliance and CPHVA (Community Practitioners and Health Visitors Association) is at http://www.nhsalliance.org/documents/clin_gov_summary.htm
- A clinical governance bibliography specifically relating to the nursing press is available from the University of Southampton at http://www.soton.ac.uk/~library/nursing/clinicalgovernance.shtml

Trusts, primary care groups and practices

Increasingly, local organisations have information on clinical governance. The following, for example, have WWW pages of relevance:

- Walsgrave Hospitals NHS Trust have clinical governance procedures at http://www.jmporter.demon.co.uk/cg/int.html
- University College London has 'Links with Clinical Governance' at http:// www.uclh.org/risk_management/links.htm
- South Manchester Primary Care Group at http://www.smanpcg.com/Subgroups/CLINICAL%20GOVERNANCE/

clingovinfo.htm and http://www. smanpcg.com/Subgroups/
CLINICAL%20GOVERNANCE/clingov.htm

Electronic journals

- *The Journal of Clinical Governance*, based at the University
  of Leicester, is at http://www.le.ac.uk/genpractice/gpaudit/
  jclingov.html

Audit

Audit is a process 'used by health professionals to assess, evaluate
and improve the care of patients in a systematic way, to enhance
their health and quality of life' (Irvine and Irvine, 1998). There
are a number of resources available for audit on the Internet. Most
clinical audit sites are found in local Trusts, although there are
useful resources on, for example, the NICE site. There is not
enough space in this chapter to discuss audit in detail, but the
resource list provides some links for you to explore.

Resource list

Email lists

Clinical audit is 'for people involved in research into, and leadership of, clinical audit in primary healthcare. The aim is to
enable exchange of information and the generation of new ideas.'
Information on this list is at http://www.mailbase.ac.uk/lists/
clinicalaudit/. Mailbase is a UK service, based at the University
of Newcastle, so the list is likely to have a UK slant.

WWW sites

- NICE on http://www.nice.org.uk/ has a clinical audit page
- Clinical Audit and Clinical Effectiveness links to a range of
  related sites via http://www.enablingpp.exec.nhs.uk/IMT/
  imtaudit.htm
- The National Centre for Clinical Audit is at http://www.
  ncca.org.uk/. 'The NCCA helps facilitate best practice in

healthcare. The Web site provides free access to the NCCA's database of resources and hosts Web pages and databases for other organisations'

- Clinical Audit Access User Group is at http://caaug. hypermart.net

Many Trusts also have pages:

- The North Staffordshire Clinical Audit Department is responsible for facilitating the audit programmes of the North Staffordshire Hospital NHS Trust and is at http://www. auditcli.demon.co.uk/homepage.htm
- South Buckinghamshire NHS Trust Clinical Effectiveness Department is at http://www.wghaudit.demon.co.uk/
- The Oxfordshire MAAG (Multidisciplinary Clinical Audit Advisory Group) is at http://www.oxmaag.demon.co.uk/html/news. htm
- 'What is Clinical Audit?' from the Royal Sussex County Hospital, Brighton, is at http://www.worthing.gov.uk/rsch/ cadept/whatis.htm
- Clinical Audit and Clinical Effectiveness from Brighton Healthcare NHS Trust on http://www.ihcd. org.uk/IMT/imtaudit.htm contains links to a range of sites dealing with clinical audit and clinical effectiveness

Clinical guidelines

The Harold Shipman case, in which the deliberate killing of well patients occurred, is certain to change the public perception of health workers. Before Shipman, there was the Beverly Allitt case, in which children were killed by a nurse in hospital. Shocking though these cases are, it is competency rather than criminality that has formed the focus in other recent events in the UK. Grave doubts have been cast on the ability of the medical profession to maintain the best clinical practice: in the scandal of the Bristol paediatric cardiac surgery unit, for example, where a much higher number of children died than in similar units elsewhere, some surgeons were disciplined. It is clear that more accountability is needed to ensure both that crimes are not committed by health professionals abusing their position of power over vulnerable patients, and that poor clinical practice is identified and dealt with.

Even prior to these cases, government policy was inevitably moving towards more accountability. The DoH has initiated NSFs, addressing high-priority areas such as mental health (NHS, 1999). These frameworks give specific guidance on what users of health-care can expect from the services. The mental health frame-work, for example, specifies the availability of services to sufferers of mental illness, as well as the agencies who should be providing the services.

The proposed National Electronic Library for Health (http://www.nelh.nhs.uk) will contain four areas, one of which is based on guidelines and audit. The site is designed to be open to both users and clinicians.

There is 'evidence of wide provincial variations in medical care' (Rappolt, 1997, pp. 977–87). Nursing, midwifery and the profes-sions allied to medicine 'are increasingly using clinical guidelines to reduce inappropriate variations in practice' (Thomas et al., 1999, pp. 40–50). These initiatives are attempts to define and specify best practice (either in overall terms through frameworks, or in detail using clinical guidelines) or to support the use of evidence-based practice by education and access to information (including for the general public). The huge increase in the number of articles on clinical guidelines is, even though there are many problems with clinical guidelines (Haycox et al., 1999; Woolf et al., 1999), evidence of the concern in the UK to make care transparent and consistent.

The DoH has issued several documents that support clinical governance and clinical guidelines (DoH, 1998a, 1999c; Mann, 1996; NHSE, 1996a, 1997b, 1998a, b, c). There are many excel-lent summaries of the issues in clinical guidelines. In the *British Medical Journal*, for example, a series of articles has been written (Baily et al., 1993; Banatvala and Doyal, 1998; Basky, 1999; Edito-rial, 1996; Emslie et al., 1993; Fairfield and Williams, 1996; Feder, 1994; Feder et al., 1995, 1999; Grol et al., 1998; Haycox et al., 1999; Heaney, 1996; Hemming and Mashford, 1993; Hurwitz, 1995; Jackson and Feder, 1998; Little et al., 1996; McColl, 1993; Mace, 1998; McNicol et al., 1993; Maisonneuve et al., 1996; Manchester, 1993; Saha, 1995; Shekelle et al., 1999; Thomson et al., 1995,

1996; West and Newton, 1997; Williams, 1999; Woolf et al., 1999). Nursing papers that have addressed the issue of clinical guidelines in the popular nursing press include '*NT*' *Learning Curve*, (1997) and *Nursing Standard* (1996). UK nursing organisations such as the RCN (1999a) have written short documents with excellent advice on how to use guidelines (RCN, 1999b).

Clinical guidelines are useful in providing a structured and evidence-based approach to specific conditions. I have interviewed many clinical nurses, mainly of F and G grades, who state that there is a problem in locating relevant guidelines. Local implementation is crucial to successful clinical guidelines, but the local guidelines should normally be based on national guidelines where available.

Guidelines are available on the Internet, and excellent documentation on the production, implementation and assessment of guidelines is available from national centres. However, in my interviews, none of the nurses was aware of these resources, despite many of them having access to the Internet at home (although few had access at work).

There is an enormous number of clinical guidelines published or available online. At the time of writing, for example, the National Guideline Clearinghouse alone contained 566 guidelines. In Scotland, the Scottish Intercollegiate Guidelines Network (1999) contained 40. Other sites of relevance include the New Zealand Guidelines Group (1999), the Canadian Medical Association (1999) and the American Medical Directors Association Clinical Practice Guidelines (AMDA, 1999).

Many guidelines will be international in nature, and there are several sites that pool guidelines from many countries into one resource. The Agency for Healthcare Policy, for example, supports research and the development of science-based clinical guidelines, performance measures and standards of quality (Clinton, 1994).

Resource list

- Agency for Healthcare Policy and Research (USA) on http://www.ahcpr.gov/
- American Medical Directors Association on http://www.amda.com/cpg/index.html

- Canadian Medical Association on http://www.cma.ca/cpgs/ index.htm
- National Electronic Library for Health (UK) on http://www. nelh.nhs.uk
- National Guideline Clearinghouse (USA) on http://www. guideline.gov/
- National Institute of Clinical Excellence (UK) on http://www. nice.org.uk/clin_guide/clingud_ind.htm
- New Zealand Guidelines Group on http://www.nzgg.org.nz/ index.htm
- Scottish Intercollegiate Guidelines Network on http://www. show.scot.nhs.uk/sign/
- Royal College of General Practitioners clinical guidelines on http: //www.rcgp.org.uk/college/activity/qualclin/guides/index.htm

CASE STUDY

In Leicester, there are acute and community Trusts. The diabetic nurse specialist based in the acute hospital wanted to develop clinical guidelines on the diabetic foot. She therefore worked with the tissue viability nurse specialist, who was based in the community Trust. By accessing the Scottish Intercollegiate Guidelines Network Web site, a relevant guideline was located (SIGN, 1997), which could be used to produce a local guideline. Furthermore, using the documentation on the Web site, the nurses were given advice on how to adapt national guidelines to local needs.

This case study shows an effective and efficient use of resources. It is labour intensive to produce guidelines, as well as being a complex process, requiring specialist skills. It is pointless to produce new guidelines where experts have already done the job nationally. It would be even more pointless to produce guidelines independently for two Trusts next door to each other. By collaborating across Trusts in a specialist area, and using as a starting point an evidence-based national guideline, a locally adapted guideline is produced that is scientific, valid and created with minimal effort.

Education

Having undergone training and qualified, most nurses had until recently little contact with education. With initiatives such as Post Registration Education and Practice, however, lifelong learning is now the norm. Thus you may be a student nurse in the course of studies, or a registered nurse undertaking a degree or higher degree, or you may be updating your skills on a short course. Even if you are not in formal education, you will be required to show evidence to the UKCC of continuing professional development with respect to updating your education. Busy nurses are increasingly accessing WWW-based material to assist in Post Registration Education and Practice or courses (many of which are part time). In addition to accessing material, nurses may use the Internet or NHSNet to communicate with and support each other. Such support could be via email or discussion groups, as well as by physical meetings, either informal or formal.

CASE STUDY

The tissue viability course in Leicester is over-subscribed. The tissue viability nurses in both Leicester Trusts (one of whom is the course coordinator) joined in discussions with the university staff to produce an online course, which can be used as a distance learning alternative to the traditional course. By linking with other Midlands universities, the course material can be offered to students in sister institutions.

In this example, efficiency is highlighted. Creating online courses is labour intensive and requires specialist skills. It is probably not cost-effective to create a course for one county. The online course will ultimately be available on the Internet to anyone with Internet access. Using this model, Leicester does not need to create all its own courses: by collaborating with other institutions, courses can be offered on a reciprocal basis or sold and purchased.

Systematic reviews

All students at any level in nursing should now be using evidence upon which to base their arguments. Their essays should therefore have reference to the current literature, and in many cases (for example, research dissertations), there should be a formal literature review. Evidence-based practice is the requirement in the clinical area, as put forward in many recent government papers, including a nursing strategy (www.doh.gov.uk/nurstrat.htm). Clinical practice will therefore have been preceded by a full review, or current practice that is based on tradition rather than evidence should be subject to a full review.

Reviews may be subjective and produced to back up rather than test the reviewer's own opinions. A high-quality review is systematic, that is, produced according to a set of rules. These will typically determine the papers to be included or excluded and the quality criteria. Thus a systematic review is more scientific than a more informal or 'narrative' review. In some cases, it is possible to combine evidence from many studies to provide greater statistical power. This is termed meta-analysis (see below).

It is not anticipated that the typical ward nurse or student will have the time or inclination to conduct a meta-analysis, and a full systematic review is labour intensive. Nursing studies are not always amenable to meta-analysis, as the studies are in many cases qualitative. However, for those subjects that do lend themselves to a meta-analysis, this will give the best basis upon which to determine the efficacy of a treatment. In all studies, a systematic review is to be preferred to a non-systematic one. While you will not be able to go into the detail offered by professional groups such as the York team discussed below, you could, however, make clear the criteria upon which you will consider a study relevant and how you will assess the quality of the study.

There are many sites offering systematic reviews of medical and nursing treatments. The time needed for one review is substantial, and your unit will need to access other centres if all clinical practice is to be evidence based. It is therefore not possible to conduct all the systematic reviews your area will need, and it may not be necessary to perform any if these are easily obtainable elsewhere.

The NHS CRD (on http://www.york.ac.uk/inst/crd/) at the University of York produces systematic reviews, and has a great deal of information on creating and finding reviews. The CRD site is so extensive that it seems superfluous to provide many further links; many of these are available from this site anyway in the 'links to related sites' from http://www.york.ac.uk/inst/crd/.

Resource list

Some of the facilities on the CRD site include:

- completed reviews on http://www.york.ac.uk/inst/crd/listcomp. htm
- reviews in progress on http://www.york.ac.uk/inst/crd/listong. htm
- training and advice on reviews on http://www.york.ac.uk/ inst/crd/training.htm
- guidelines for those carrying out or commissioning reviews on http://www.york.ac.uk/inst/crd/report4.htm. This is a large document with extensive information on how the CRD carries out its own reviews, which is an excellent resource for those wishing to review studies themselves
- finding studies for systematic reviews on http://www.york.ac. uk/inst/crd/revs.htm
- databases that you can search for reviews on http://nhscrd. york.ac.uk/welcome.html including the Database of Abstracts of Reviews of Effectiveness

Electronic journals or journals available on the Internet

- The Centre for Evidence-based Medicine on http://cebm.jr2. ox.ac.uk/ from which you can access *Bandolier,* a newsletter of evidence-based medicine and healthcare
- The Effective Healthcare bulletin on http://www.york.ac.uk/ inst/crd/ehcb.htm is the journal that publishes reviews from the CRD

CASE STUDY

In a community hospital for the elderly, falls are common. A reason for admission is falling, or a diagnosis known as 'off legs', which means that the patient is, for whatever reason, not able to mobilise independently. I was asked by the sister for any information on falls or guidelines on the prevention of falls. A search found a systematic review of falls published by the CRD. The sister used this review to inform ward practice, with a view to creating local guidelines in due course.

Meta-analysis

The number of articles on meta-analysis has increased substantially over the past 10 years. For an excellent overview of the progression of this discipline, and some practical methods of completing a meta-analysis, see the the *British Medical Journal's* 1997 series of seven articles, at least five of which are available in full text (see the resource list). There are many links in these articles to other articles, some of them available freely as full text over the Web. While the titles appear to be highly technical, the information is in fact accessible and very relevant to nursing. This is an area that is very important, but most clinical nurses will not be engaged in a meta-analysis, so it will not be discussed further here.

Resource list

- http://www.bmj.com/cgi/content/full/315/7121/1533 Meta-analysis: principles and procedures
- http://www.bmj.com/cgi/content/full/316/7124/61 Meta-analysis bias in location and selection of studies
- http://www.bmj.com/cgi/content/full/316/7125/140 Meta-analysis, spurious precision? Meta-analysis of observational studies
- http://www.bmj.com/cgi/content/full/316/7126/221 Meta-analysis: unresolved issues and future developments
- http://www.bmj.com/cgi/content/full/315/7122/1610 Meta-analysis: beyond the grand mean?

Hospital information support systems

HISSs have been implemented in many clinical areas, typically acute hospitals. These provide integrated information available from many different units. Pathology results and nursing clinical notes are available to authorised users via these systems. The systems are clinically based and provide information that assists in caring for patients, in contradistinction to patient administration systems, which are designed for administrative information such as bed occupancy. A HISS may form the basis for electronic patient records.

CASE STUDY

Nutrition is highly relevant to wound healing, particularly to pressure sores. There are many studies that appear to show that low albumin in particular is related to the later occurrence of pressure sores. There is, however, a problem in that pressure sores can themselves lower the albumin level as it is lost from the wound surface. So does low albumin cause sores, or does having a sore cause low albumin? Studies accessed via Medline (in this case from the Web, although there are other methods, via CD-ROM for example) were inconclusive and contradictory. I wanted to do a prospective study in which patients with no sores were followed up to see whether they developed sores. This would be expensive, and I could only obtain moderate funding.

A contact at Queen's Hospital, Burton, where a HISS system is in place, informed me that serum albumin, Waterlow scores and data on the presence of sores are routinely collected on admission, and the later occurrence of sores is recorded. This gave the nearly optimal data set for a prospective study, which was later carried out in collaboration with the tissue viability nurse and the clinical pathologist from the Queen's Hospital (Anthony et al., 2000).

This case study shows how one may, if the data are appropriate, use data collected for clinical purposes for a research study. This is a very efficient use of resources. You should note that ethical approval was still required for this study as the data were collected for clinical purposes and could not therefore automatically be used for another purpose. What was particularly useful in this study was that the data were already collected on a computer system, and they were downloaded onto a spreadsheet. The study then consisted of analysing the data and writing the study, rather than collecting the data.

One disadvantage with this approach is that the data collected for clinical purposes are rarely ideal for research purposes. In this case, the data were sufficiently close to my needs for me to be able to use the HISS data. I would ideally have liked the Waterlow scores split by sub-score (there are 11 sub-scores, but all the HISS system reported was the total). However, discussions with a local Trust indicated that they would be able to start collecting these data on their HISS.

Care plans

There are surprisingly few Web sites devoted to care plans or with care plans available. This is in sharp distinction to the sites devoted to clinical guidelines, on which a huge number of guidelines are available.

What is evident here is a lack of evidence for the basis underlying the care plans. The care plans are simply given as procedures to follow, with no references or links to more detailed information. This contrasts strongly with the clinical guidelines sites, where there is typically extensive detail on the science behind the guidelines and clear indications on how the guidelines were developed and validated.

Resource list

There is an email list, CAREPL-L (CAREPL-L@LISTSERV.ACSU. BUFFALO.EDU) and archives of this list are on http://listserv. acsu.buffalo.edu/archives/carepl-l.html, including care plans sent in to the list.

WWW sites include the following:

- links to nursing care plans and case studies on http://www. lib.iun.indiana.edu/careplan.htm which contains links, software and case studies
- the Careplan Resource Center on http://www.careplans.com/
- care plan guidelines on http://home.hiwaay.net/~theholt1/ NURS1100/careplan.htm is part of a nursing course and gives some information on creating care plans
- care planning on http://dmoz.org/Health/Nursing/Care_ Planning/ which has specific care plans on http://www. aofm.com/home/health/care_plans/. There is, for example, a care plan for pressure sores on http://www.aofm.com/ homehealth/care_plans/plan10.htm
- Computer Programs and Systems, Inc. has http://www. cpsinet.com/system2000/careplans.shtml which is a computer company site creating modules for care plans
- nursing care plans are included among other material on http://www.lopez1.com/lopez/nursing.students/care.plans.htm

- Mercy Health Plans on http://www.carechoices.com/ has some guidelines on, for example, adult male preventive health screens
- NIT on http://nursesintraining.8m.com/careplan.htm has many care plans and links

Patient information

It would seem an obvious use of the Web to allow patients to access information on their care. Some Trusts do provide information, but this is not uniform. One document discussing patient information is *Patient Information – A Trustwide Approach from Stockport Healthcare NHS Trust* on http://www.centreforhiq. demon.co.uk/newsletter/nl4d.htm.

The provision of patient information is an important use of the Internet, and is one of the aims of the government as stated in *Information for Health* (NHSE, 1998).

Resource list

Patient information sites

- The Centre for Health Information Quality on http://www. centreforhiq.demon.co.uk/ was launched in November 1997 as part of the Patient Partnership Strategy, a UK NHS initiative
- The Patient Education Institute on http://www.patient-education.com/ publishes interactive patient education software
- The Patient Advocate on http://www.thepatientadvocate.com/ was developed as an educational and consulting medium
- Choices Women's Medical Center on http://gynpages.com/ choices/index.html is a comprehensive ambulatory medical facility that has been run by women since 1971

Patient information on specific diseases

- The Patient Advocate Foundation on http://www. patientadvocate.org/ provides education and legal counselling to cancer patients concerning managed care, insurance and financial issues

- Contemporary Health Communications on http://patient-info.com/ provides plastic, reconstructive and cosmetic surgeons with patient information brochures and the Patient Information Network
- LocateAnEyeDoc.com on http://patient.isrs.org/ is a guide to laser vision correction. Moorfields (Eye) Hospital on http://www.moorfields.org.uk/ has general information; specifically, their mobile unit is on http://www.moorfields.org.uk/mobile-unit.html
- The International Myeloma Foundation on http://myeloma.org/Seminars.html conducts an ongoing series of educational seminars, primarily for patients and their families
- Information for Cancer Patients and their Families on http://www.icr.ac.uk/careinfo.htm includes a large list of cancer patient information sites, for example Patient Information Publications on http://www.patient.org.uk/ plus many specific cancer sites

Sites with links

Patient Information Publications have UK Self-help and Patient Groups Web Links on http://www.patient.org.uk/index.htm. For example under 'Elderly Support' they include:

- Age Concern England on http://www.ace.org.uk/
- Age Resource on http://www.ace.org.uk/ageres/default.htm
- the Alzheimer's Disease Society on http://www.alzheimers.org.uk/
- Alzheimer's Scotland – Action on Dementia on http://www.alzscot.org/
- the Dementia Care Trust on http://www.dct.org.uk/
- Different Strokes on http://www.strokes.demon.co.uk/
- Help the Aged on http://www.helptheaged.org.uk/

They also list contact details of further groups and organisations without Web sites.

The Health Centre on http://www.healthcentre.org.uk/hc/clinic/websites/default.htm guides you through the huge amount of medical and health information from the UK that is available on the Internet.

International sites

- A Spanish site concerning Alzheimer's disease is available on http://www.solitel.es/alzheimer/indexi.htm
- A German patient information site on http://www.patient.de/ is written in both the native language and English

Electronic journals

- *Signpost* on http://signpostjournal.connect-2.co.uk/ is a specialist quarterly journal aimed at those working with and caring for people with dementia, older people with mental health problems, and their carers

Assessment of information

Obtaining information from the Internet is potentially problematic. Many authors have expressed concern over, for example, patients obtaining information from non-authorised sites, where the quality of the information may be suspect. This is, however, not a new problem. You could, for example, question whether an article in a magazine or tabloid newspaper is as evidence based as an academic article in a professional journal. You could also ask whether patients talk to other patients about their condition and what information they might get.

It is more constructive to provide patients with appropriate information. If patients come armed with information obtained from the Web, you should not dismiss them but instead assess the quality based on sensible criteria. For a good discussion of how you might do this, you can read Peter Murray's article available online at http://www.nursing-standard.co.uk/archives/vol11-45/ol-art.htm suggesting we should be concerned with:

- the *authority* of the author or creator (which includes the author being identified)
- the *currency* or updatedness, and stability of the information
- the *accuracy* of the information and its comparability with related sources

- its *workability* in terms of user-friendliness, connectivity and search access
- the *purpose* of the resource

Murray concludes that the quality of Web-based resources varies greatly, and while new assessment criteria are needed, 'the five traditional print criteria of accuracy, authority, objectivity, currency, coverage may be appropriate'.

Conclusion

There is an enormous amount of assistance that IT can give the working nurse, including HISSs, electronic patient records and tele-medicine. The systems you find will vary from hospital to hospital. The Web-based information systems will, however, be similar whether you access them from home, at work via a LAN with access to the Internet, or through NHSNet. This chapter has offered some of these resources, with special reference to clinical guidelines and clinical governance.

Exercises

- You are an F-grade sister (a head nurse in the USA). A patient is admitted to your ward with a severe cerebrovascular accident (which occurred three months ago) for rehabilitation. She has made very little progress with intensive physiotherapy, which has been reduced from daily to weekly. She suffers from central pain and is being treated with a tricyclic antidepressant. Her daughter visits and asks to see you, bringing with her a sheet of information from netdoctor (a Web site) on the antidepressant, a page from the British Stroke Association's Web page with information on physiotherapy in cerebrovascular accident, and a Web page suggesting that seaweed is useful for stroke patients' pain. She wants to know why her mother is on the antidepressant medication regime and why the frequency of the physiotherapy is being reduced. The daughter asks whether seaweed is used in your ward. What advice could you offer her, and what resources might you find useful in this context?

- You have taken up a new post, Head of Quality, for your Trust, an orthopaedic surgical hospital. You are told that there is a high level of pressure sores in the hospital, especially on the trauma ward. What action might you take to investigate?

- You are a practice development nurse at a small community hospital. At a unit meeting, one of your colleagues, a staff nurse who works in a ward where many elderly patients are sent for convalescence, states that she knows of no guidelines for treating leg ulcers. You can locate none in your Trust. How might you locate a guideline and implement it locally?

- You are undertaking a part-time degree in nursing. For your dissertation, you have selected a problem area in your Trust, the security of nursing staff, several attacks having been made on nurses in recent months. Discuss how you might conduct a systematic review of the subject. What online resources might you find useful?

- You are asked to produce a care plan for depression in your unit. How might you locate a pre-existing care plan to give you some suggestions? How would you assess the validity of such a care plan? What alternatives to care plans could you suggest?

Key Point Summary

- Nurses do not need to understand computing; they need to understand information

- Information systems vary from hospital to hospital

- The World Wide Web (WWW) is similar from wherever you access it

- There are many WWW resources that are useful to clinical nurses

- Clinical governance is well served by the WWW

- Clinical guidelines are available on the WWW

Note

1. If you are involved in training, you may find the following resources useful: *Learning to Manage Health Information* (NHS Executive, 1999), *Assessing the Impact of LIS on IM&T* (NHS Information Authority, 1999b) and *Training Needs Analysis* (NHS Information Authority, 1999c).

References

Abdel-Halim, A.A. (1983) Power equalization, participative decision-making and individual differences. *Human Relations* **36**(18): 683–704.

Abdellah, B. and Levine, E. (1957) Polling patients and personnel. Part 1: When patients say about their nursing care. *Hospitals* **31**: 44–88.

Abel-Smith, B. (1964) *The Hospitals 1800–1948*. London: Heinemann.

Akinsanya, J. (1985) Learning about life. *Senior Nurse* **2**(5): 24–5

AMDA (American Medical Directors Association (1999) *AMDA Clinical Practice Guidelines*. Columbia, MD: AMDA.

Anderson, J. and Elfert, H. (1989) Managing chronic illness in the family: women as caretakers. *Journal of Advanced Nursing* **14**: 735–43.

Anthony, D.M. (1996) *Health on the Internet*. Oxford: Blackwell Scientific.

Anthony, D., Reynolds, T. and Russell, L. (2000) An investigation into the use of serum albumin in pressure sore prediction. *Journal of Advanced Nursing* **32**(2): 359–65.

Ashley, J.A. (1980) Power in structured misogyny: implications for the politics of care. *Advances in Nursing Science* **2**(3): 3–22.

Audit Commission (1993) *Children First: A Study of Hospital Services*. London: HMSO.

Audit Commission Report (1996) *Form Follows Function*. Oxford: Audit Commission Publications.

Bachrach, P. and Baratz, M. (1962) Power and domination in British society. In Dearlove, J. and Saunders, P. (eds) (1984) *Introduction to British Politics*. Cambridge: Polity Press.

Baily, G.G., Hammer, M.R., Hanley, S.P., Pattrick, M.G. and De Kretser, D.M. (1993) Implementing clinical guidelines. Computers allow instant access [letter]. *British Medical Journal* **307**(6905): 679.

Baldwin, S. (1999) Care in the community for people with a learning disability: choice, opportunity and risk. *Mental Healthcare* **2**(5): 167–9.

Banatvala, N. and Doyal, L. (1998) Knowing when to say 'no' on the student elective. Students going on electives abroad need clinical guidelines [editorial]. *British Medical Journal* **316**(7142): 1404–5.

Basky, G. (1999) Doctors resist adopting clinical guidelines [news]. *British Medical Journal* **318**(7195): 1370.

Bennis, W. (1985) *Leaders.* Toronto: Harper & Row.

Bennis, W. (1993) *An Invented Life.* London: Century.

Bernarde, M.A. and Mayerson, E.W. (1978) Patient–physician negotiation. *Journal of the American Medical Association* **239**: 1413–15.

Biley, F. (1992) Some determinants that affect patient participation in decision-making about nursing care. *Journal of Advanced Nursing* **17**: 414–21.

Binnie, A. and Titchen, A. (1998) *Patient-centred Nursing. An Action Research Study of Practice Development in Acute Medical Unit.* Report No. 18. Oxford: RCN.

Bircumshaw, D. (1990) The utilisation of research findings in clinical nursing practice. *Journal of Advanced Nursing* **15**: 1272–80.

Bishop, V. (1994) Clinical supervision for an accountable profession. *Nursing Times* **90**(39): 34–9.

Bishop, V. (1998) Clinical supervision, what is it? In Bishop V. (ed.) *Clinical Supervision in Practice: Some Questions, Answers and Guidelines.* Basingstoke/London: Macmillan/NTResearch.

Bishop, V. (1999) Surviving a research degree: a personal view and review of the literature. In Bishop, V. (ed.) *Working Towards a Research Degree: Insights from the Nursing Perspective.* London: NTBooks.

Bishop, V. and Butterworth, T. (1994) *Clinical Supervision: A Report of the Trust Nurse Executive Workshops.* Leeds: NHSE.

Blackman, P.S. (2000) *Exclusion by Default* [conference paper]. Leicester: Mary Seacole Research Centre.

Boden, L. and Kelly, D. (1999) Clinical governance: the route to (modern, dependable) nursing research? *Nursing Times Research* **4**(3): 177–88.

Bonnell, C. (1999) Evidence-based nursing: a stereotyped view of quantitative and experimental research could work against professional autonomy and authority. *Journal of Advanced Nursing* **30**(1): 18–23.

Breakwell, G.M., Hammond, S. and Fife-Schaw, C. (1995) *Research Methods in Psychology.* London: Sage.

Brindle, D. (1996) Back to basics of the bar. *Guardian*, Society Supplement, 24 July, p. 11.

Brownlea, A., Taylor, C., Landbeck, M., Wishart, R., Nalder, G. and Behan, S. (1980) Cited in Wade, S. (1995) Partnership in care: a critical review. *Nursing Standard* **9**(48): 333–5.

Burns, N. and Grove, S.K. (1987) *The Practice of Nursing Research. Conduct, Critique and Utilisation.* Philadelphia: W.B. Saunders.

Butterworth, A. (1998) The potential of clinical supervision for nurses, midwives and health visitors. In Bishop, V. (ed.) *Clinical*

Supervision in Practice: Some Questions, Answers and Guidelines. Basingstoke/London: Macmillan/NTResearch.

Butterworth, A.C. and Bishop, V.A. (1995) Identifying the characteristics of optimum practice: findings from a survey of practice experts in nursing, midwifery and health visiting. *Journal of Advanced Nursing* **22**: 24–32.

Butterworth, C., Carson, J., White, E., Jeacock, J., Clements, A. and Bishop, V. (1996a) *It's Good to Talk? The 23 Site Evaluation Project of Clinical Supervision in England and Scotland. An Interim Report.* Manchester: Manchester University.

Butterworth, T. (1992) Clinical supervision as an emerging idea in nursing. In Butterworth, T. and Faugier, J. (eds) *Clinical Supervision and Mentorship in Nursing.* London: Chapman & Hall.

Butterworth, T. (1996) Primary attempts at research-based evaluation of clinical supervision. *Nursing Times Research* **1**(2): 96–101.

Butterworth, T. (1998) Review. *Nursing Times Research* **3**(2): 151.

Butterworth, T., Bishop, V. and Carson, J. (1996b) First steps towards evaluating clinical supervision in nursing. Part 1: Theory, policy and practice development. A review. *Journal of Clinical Nursing* **5**: 127–32.

Calman, K. and Hine, D. (1995) *A Policy Framework for Commissioning Cancer Services.* London: DoH.

Campbell, A. (1984) *Moderated Love – a Theology of Professional Care.* SPCK: London.

Canadian Medical Association. Accessed 21-11-1999 http://www.cma.ca/cpgs/index.htm.

Carr-Hill, R. and Drew, D. (1988) Blacks, police and crime. In Bhat, P. (ed.) *Britain's Black Population.* Aldershot: Gower.

Carson, D. (1995) *Mental Handicap Research.* Kidderminster: BILD Publications.

Casey, A. (1988) A partnership with child and family. *Senior Nurse* **8**(4): 8–9.

Champion, V. and Leach, A. (1989) Variables related to research utilisation in nursing: an empirical investigation. *Journal of Advanced Nursing* **14**: 705–10.

Chater, S. (1975) *Understanding Research in Nursing.* Geneva: WHO.

Christensen, J. (1993) *Nursing Partnership – a Model for Nursing Practice.* London: Churchill Livingstone.

Clinton, J.J. (1994) Enhancing clinical-practice – the role of practice guidelines. *American Psychologist* **49**(1): 30–3.

Closs, J. and Cheater, F.M. (1996) Audit or research – what is the difference? *Journal of Clinical Nursing* **5**: 249–57.

Closs, J. and Cheater, F.M. (1999) Evidence for nursing practice: a clarification of the issues. *Journal of Advanced Nursing* **30**(1): 10–17.

Coombes, R. and Green, K. (1989) Work organisation and product change in the service sector. In Wood, S. (ed.) *The Transformation of Work*. London: Unwin Hyman.

Coombs, M. (1999) Building bridges between nursing research and practice. In Bishop, V. (ed.) *Working Towards a Research Degree, Insights from the Nursing Perspective*. London: NTBooks.

Dahl, R.A. (1961) *Who Governs?* New Haven, CT: Yale University Press.

Darbyshire, P. (1994) *Living with a Sick Child in Hospital*. London: Chapman & Hall.

Davies, D. (1995) *Gender and the Professional Predicament in Nursing*. Milton Keynes: Open University Press.

Dearlove, J. and Saunders, P. (1984) *Introduction to British Politics*. Cambridge: Polity Press.

DoH (Department of Health) (1989a) *A Strategy for Nursing*. London: HMSO.

DoH (Department of Health) (1989b) *Working for Patients*. London: DoH.

DoH (Department of Health) (1989c) *Caring for People. Community Care in the Next Decade and Beyond*. Cmnd 840. London: HMSO.

DoH (Department of Health) (1990) *Working for Patients*. London: DoH.

DoH (Department of Health) (1991a) *The Patient's Charter*. London: HMSO.

DoH (Department of Health) (1991b) *Welfare of Children and Young People in Hospital*. London: HMSO.

DoH (Department of Health) (1993a) *Report of the Taskforce on the Strategy for Nursing, Midwifery and Health Visitors*. London: DoH.

DoH (Department of Health (1993b) *Hospital Doctors: Training for the Future*. Report of the Working Group on Specialist Medical Training (The Calman Report). London: DoH.

DoH (Department of Health) (1995) *The Nursing and Therapy Professions' Contribution to Health Services Research and Development* (The Calman Hine Report). London: DoH.

DoH (Department of Health) (1996) *The Patient's Charter and You*. London: DoH.

DoH (Department of Health) (1998) *Clinical Governance: Quality in the New NHS*. London: DoH.

DoH (Department of Health) (1998a) *A First Class Service: Quality in the New NHS*. Wetherby: DoH, www.doh.gov.uk/newnhs/qualsum.htm

DoH (Department of Health) (1998b) *The New NHS: Modern, Dependable*. London: DoH Crown Copyright.

DoH (Department of Health) (1999) *Modernising Health and Social Services: Developing the Workforce*. HSC.199999/111. LAC(99)18. London: DoH.

DoH (Department of Health) (1999a) *Making a Difference. Strengthening the Nursing, Midwifery and Health Visiting Contribution to Health and Healthcare.* London: DoH.

DoH (Department of Health) (1999b) *National Service Framework for Mental Health. Modern Standards and Service Models.* London: DoH.

DoH (Department of Health) (1999c) *Steps Towards Clinical Governance.* London: DoH.

DoH (Department of Health) (2000a) *National Service Framework for Coronary Heart Disease. Modern Standards and Service Models.* London: DoH.

DoH (Department of Health) (2000b) *A Health Service for all Talents: Developing the NHS Workforce.* A Consultation Document on the Review of Workforce Planning. London: DoH.

DHSS (Department of Health and Social Security) (1980) *Inequalities in Health: Report of a Research Working Group* (The Black Report). London: DHSS.

Dix, T. and Gilbert, T. (1995) Care in the community for people with a learning disability: choice, opportunity and risk. *Mental Healthcare* **2**(5): 167–9.

Dooley, F. (1999) The named nurse in practice. *Nursing Standard* **13**(34): 33–8.

Driscoll, J. (2000) *Practicing Clinical Supervision: A Reflective Approach.* London: Baillière Tindall/RCN.

Duffy, M.E. (1985) Designing nursing research: the qualitative–quantitative debate. *Journal of Advanced Nursing* **10**: 225–32.

Dunn, C. and Bishop, V. (1998) Clinical supervision: its implementation in one acute sector. In Bishop, V. (ed.) *Clinical Supervision in Practice: Some Questions, Answers and Guidelines.* Basingstoke/London: Macmillan/NTResearch.

Dworkin, G. (1988) *The Theory and Practice of Autonomy.* Cambridge: Cambridge University Press.

Dyer, A.R. and Blosch, S. (1987) Informed consent and the psychiatric patient. *Journal of Medical Ethics* **13**: 12–15.

Editorial (1996) Clinical guidelines in the independent healthcare sector. *British Medical Journal* **312**: 1554–5.

Elliott, M.A and Turrell, A.R. (1996) Dilemmas for the empowering nurse. *Journal of Nursing Management* **4**: 273–9.

Emslie, C., Grimshaw, J. and Templeton, A. (1993) Do clinical guidelines improve general practice management and referral of infertile couples? *British Medical Journal* **306**(6894): 1728–31.

Fairfield, G. and Williams, R. (1996) Clinical guidelines in the independent healthcare sector. *British Medical Journal* **312**(7046): 1554–5.

Faugier, J. and Butterworth, T. (1994) *Clinical Supervision. A Position Paper.* Manchester: Manchester University.

Feder, G. (1994) Clinical guidelines in 1994. *British Medical Journal* **309**(6967): 1457–8.

Feder, G., Griffiths, C., Highton, C., Eldridge, S., Spence, M. and Southgate, L. (1995) Do clinical guidelines introduced with practice based education improve care of asthmatic and diabetic patients? A randomised controlled trial in general practices in east London. *British Medical Journal* **311**(7018): 1473–8.

Feder, G., Eccles, M., Grol, R., Griffiths, C. and Grimshaw, J. (1999) Clinical guidelines: using clinical guidelines. *British Medical Journal* **318**(7185): 728–30.

Fenton S. (1989) Racism is harmful to your health. In Cox, J. and Bodstock, S.J. (eds) *Racial Discrimination in the Health Service.* Keele: Keele University.

Foucault, M. (1980) *Power Knowledge.* Horrocks.

Fox, N.J. (1999) *Beyond Health, Postmodernism and Embodiment.* London: Free Association Books.

French, P. (1999) The development of evidence based nursing. *Journal of Advanced Nursing* **29**(1): 72–8.

Freshwater, D. (1999) Taking responsibility for making a difference. *Nursing Times Research* **4**(5): 395.

Freshwater, D. (2000) Research and the reflective practitioner. In Rolfe, G., Freshwater, D. and Jasper, M. (eds) *Critical Reflection for Nursing and the Helping Professions: A Users Guide.* London: Macmillan.

Gadd, D., McFadden, K. and Colgan, L. (1995) *Research Based Care Planning: A Case Study of Research used by Mental Health Nurses.* Manchester: Cartmel NDU.

Gibbs, I. (1991) Parents as partners in care. *Paediatric Nursing* **8**(6): 24–7.

Gibson, C. (1991) A concept analysis of empowerment. *Journal of Advanced Nursing* **16**: 354–61.

Glover, D. (1999) Accountability. Nursing Times Monograph. London: Emap Publications.

GMC (General Medical Council) (1995) *Good Medical Practice.* London: GMC.

Greenwood, J. (1984) Nursing research: a position paper. *Journal of Advanced Nursing* **9**: 77–82.

Grol, R., Dalhuijsen, J., Thomas, S., Veld, C., Rutten, G. and Mokkink, H. (1998) Attributes of clinical guidelines that influence use of guidelines in general practice: observational study. *British Medical Journal* **317**(7162): 858–61.

Hague, D. (1993) *Transforming the Dinosaurs.* Demos: London.

Ham, C. (1992) *Health Policy in Britain,* 3rd edn. London: Macmillan.

Hammer, M. (1993) *The Process Oriented Organisation.* Unpublished document.

Hammer, M. and Champy, J. (1993) *Reengineering the Corporation.* London: Nicholas Brearley.

Hancock, C. (2000) Plenary keynote paper, RCN Research Society Conference, Sheffield.

Hancock, H.C. (1997) Professional responsibility: implications for nursing practice within the realms of cardiothoracics. *Journal of Advanced Nursing* **25**: 1054–60.

Handy, C. (1994) *The Empty Raincoat. Making Sense of the Future.* London: Hutchinson.

Hanson. J.L. (1994) Advanced practice nurse's application of the Stetler model for research utilisation in improving bereavement care. *Oncology Nursing Forum* **21**(4): 720–4.

Harrison, S., Hunter, D., Marnoch, G. and Pollitt, C. (1992) *Just Managing: Power and the Culture in the National Health Service.* London: Macmillan.

Hart, G.M. (1982) *The Process of Clinical Evaluation.* Baltimore, MD: University Press.

Haycox, A., Bagust, A. and Walley, T. (1999) Clinical guidelines – the hidden costs. *British Medical Journal* **318**(7180): 391–3.

Heaney, D. (1996) Clinical guidelines may obviate need for thought [letter, comment]. *British Medical Journal* **312**(7032): 706.

Hemming, M. and Mashford, M.L. (1993) Implementing clinical guidelines. It works in Australia. *British Medical Journal* **307**(6905): 678.

Henneman, E.A., Lee, J.L. and Cohen, J.I. (1995) Collaboration: a concept analysis. *Journal of Advanced Nursing* **21**: 103–9.

Heyman, B. and Huckle, S. (1993) Normal life in a hazardous world: how adults with a moderate learning disability and their carers cope with risks and dangers. *Disability, Handicap and Society* **8**(2): 143–59.

Hill, Y.W. (1996) Children in intensive care: can nurse–parent partnership enable the child and family to cope more effectively? *Intensive and Critical Care* **12**: 155–60.

Hippocrates Cited in Kornfield, D.S. (1972) The hospital environment: its impact on the patient. *Advanced Psychosomatic Medicine* **8**: 252–70.

Hoskins, C.K. (1998) *Developing Research in Nursing and Health. Quantitative and Qualitative Methods.* New York: Springer.

Hughson, E.A. and Brown, R.I. (1988) The evaluation of rehabilitation programmes. *Irish Journal of Psychology* **9**(2): 249–63.

Hull, C. and Redfern, L. (1996) *Profiles and Portfolios.* Basingstoke: Macmillan.

Hunt, M. (1987) The process of translating research findings into nursing practice. *Journal of Advanced Nursing* **6**: 189–94.

174   *References*

Hurwitz, B. (1995) Clinical guidelines and the law. *British Medical Journal* **311**(7019): 1517–18.

Irvine, D. and Irvine, S. (1998) *Making Sense of Audit*. Abingdon: Radcliffe Medical Press.

Jackson, R. and Feder, G. (1998) Guidelines for clinical guidelines. *British Medical Journal* **317**(7156): 427–8.

Jacobs, K.D. (1980) Does the nurse practitioner involve the patient in his care. *Nursing Outlook* **28**(8): 501–5.

Jewell, S. (1994) Patient participation: what does it mean to nurses? *Journal of Advanced Nursing* **19**: 433–8.

Johnson, S. (1995) Pathway to the heart of quality care. *Nursing Management* **1**(8): 26–7.

Johnston, C. (1999a) Board editorial. *Nursing Times Research* **4**(1): 404.

Johnston, C. (1999b) Trust nurse directors can lead the way in nursing's bid for a bigger slice of the resource cake [guest editorial]. *Nursing Times Research* **4**(6): 404.

Jones, H. (1996) Autonomy and paternalism: partners or rivals? *British Journal of Nursing* **5**(6): 378–81.

Jowett, S., Peters, M. and Wilson-Barnett, J. (1999) The impact of Scope – practitioners' views on its relevance and potential for service development. *Nursing Times Research* **4**(6): 422–31.

Kawik, L. (1995) A descriptive study to explore the perceptions of nurse and parents in relation to parental participation and partnership in caring for a hospitalised child. Unpublished Masters Dissertation, University of Reading.

Keill, P. and Johnson, T. (1994) Optimizing performance through process improvement. *Nursing Care Quality* **9**.

Kennerfalk, L. and Klefsjø, B. (1995) A change process for adapting organizations to a total quality management strategy. *Total Quality Management* **6**(2).

Kets De Vries, M. (1993) *The Leadership Mystique*. Working papers. Paris: INSEAD.

Kohner, N. (1994) *Clinical Supervision in Practice*. London: King's Fund.

Kyzer, D. (1992) Nursing policy; the supply and demand for nurses. In Robinson, J., Gray, A. and Elkan, R. (eds) *Policy Issues in Nursing*. Milton Keynes: Open University Press.

Lacey, E.A. (1994) Research utilisation in research practice: a pilot study. *Journal of Advanced Nursing* **19**: 987–95.

Lathlean, J. (1992) The contribution of lecturer practitioners to theory and practice in nursing. *Journal of Clinical Nursing* **1**: 231–42.

Le May, A., Mulhall, A. and Alexander, C. (1998) Bridging the research–practice gap: exploring the research cultures of practitioners and managers. *Journal of Advanced Nursing* **28**(2): 428–37.

Light, D. (1999) *Future Challenges for the NHS: An International Perspective on the 50th Anniversary.* London: Nuffield Trust.

Link Up (1999) (RCN) (February) pp. 3–5.

Little, P., Smith, L., Cantrell, T., Chapman, J., Langridge, J. and Pickering, R. (1996) General practitioners' management of acute back pain: a survey of reported practice compared with clinical guidelines. *British Medical Journal* **312**: 485–88.

Littlewood, J. (1989) A model for nursing using anthropological literature. *Nursing Standard* **26**: 221–9.

Long, A.F. (1998) Health services research – a radical approach to cross the research and development divide. In Baker, M. and Kirk, S. (eds) *Research and Development for the NHS.* Oxford: Radcliffe Medical Press.

Lukes, S. (1974) *Power – A Radical View.* London: Macmillan.

Luthera, M. (1988) Race, community housing and the State: an historical overview. In Bhat, P. (ed.) *Britain's Black Population.* Aldershot: Gower.

MacCarthy, B. and Craissati, J. (1989) Ethnic differences in response to adversity: a community sample of Bangladeshis and their indigenous neighbours. *Social Psychiatry and Social Epidemiology* **24**(4): 196–201.

Mace, C.J. (1998) Prognosis of symptoms that are medically unexplained. Clinical guidelines are needed [letter]. *British Medical Journal* **317**(7157): 536.

Macpherson Report (1999) *The Stephen Lawrence Inquiry; Report of an Inquiry by Sir William Macpherson.* Cmd 4262. London: HMSO.

McCaugherty, D. (1991) The use of a teaching model to promote reflection and the experiential integration of theory and practice in first year student nurses: an action research study. *Journal of Advanced Nursing* **16**: 534–43.

McColl, A. (1993) Implementing clinical guidelines. Guidelines may not be cost effective. *British Medical Journal* **307**(6905): 678–9.

McMahon, R. (1986) Nursing as therapy. *Professional Nurse* **1**(10): 270–2.

McNicol, M., Layton, A. and Morgan, G. (1993) Implementing clinical guidelines has a lot to offer patient care [letter]. *British Medical Journal* **307**(6905): 678.

McSkimming, S. (1996) Creating a cultural norm for research and research utilisation in a clinical agency. *Western Journal of Nursing Research* **18**: 606–11.

Mahood, N.J., Colgan, L.M. and Bocus, Y. (1995) Training needs analysis of qualified nurses. Unpublished report, NHS Trust, Mental Health Services of Salford.

176   *References*

Maisonneuve, H., Colin, C. and Matillon, Y. (1996) French regulatory medical references are criteria, not clinical guidelines [letter, comment]. *British Medical Journal* **313**(7060): 818.

Malin, N. and Teasdale, K. (1991) Caring versus empowerment: considerations for nursing practice. *Journal of Advanced Nursing* **16**: 657–62.

Manchester, D. (1993) Neuroleptics, learning-disability, and the community – some history and mystery. *British Medical Journal* **307**(6897): 184–7.

Mann, T. (1996) *Clincal Guidelines: Using Clinical Guidelines To Improve Patient Care Within the NHS.* Leeds: NHSE.

Marks-Maran, D. (1999) Reconstructing nursing: evidence, artistry and the curriculum. *Nurse Education Today* **19**: 3–11.

Masterclass (1998) *Nursing Times Research* **3**(4): 289–90.

Masterson, A. and Maslin-Prothero, S. (1999) *Nursing and Politics – Power Through Practice.* London: Churchill Livingston.

Melia, K.M. (1989) *Everyday Nursing Ethics.* Basingstoke: Macmillan.

Miller, W.L. and Crabtree, B.F. (1999) Overview of qualitative research. In Crabtree, B.F. and Miller, W.L. (eds) *Doing Qualitative Research,* 2nd edn. London: Sage.

Mishler, E. (1979) Meaning in content: is there any other kind? *Harvard Educational Review* **49**: 1–19.

Moores, Y. (1999) Making a difference – the foundation for a future ripe with opportunity [guest editorial]. *Nursing Times Research* **4**(6): 405.

NHS (National Health Service) (1999) *Modern Standards and Service Models. Mental Health: National Service Frameworks.* London: DoH.

NHSE (National Health Service Executive) (1994a) *NHS-wide Networking and Acute Units: A Briefing.* London: NHSE.

NHSE (National Health Service Executive) (1994b) *NHS-wide Networking for FHSAs – Moving Together.* London: NHSE.

NHSE (National Health Service Executive) (1994c) *A Strategy for NHS-wide Networking.* London: NHSE.

NHSE (National Health Service Executive) (1995) *NHS-wide Networking Programme: NHS Wide Networking – Security Project. Security Guide for IM&T Specialists.* London: NHSE.

NHSE (National Health Service Executive) (1996a) *Promoting Clinical Effectiveness: A Framework for Action in and Through the NHS.* Leeds: NHSE.

NHSE (National Health Service Executive) (1996b) *Guidelines for Security Audits in the National Health Service.* London: NHSE.

NHSE (National Health Service Executive) (1997a) *A Survey of Acute Hospital Patient Centred and Clinical Information Systems.* London: NHSE.

NHSE (National Health Service Executive) (1997b) *Clinical Effectiveness Resource Pack.* Wetherby: NHSE.
NHSE (National Health Service Executive) (1998) *Research: What's in it for Consumers?* London: DoH.
NHSE (National Health Service Executive) (1998a) *Information for Health. An Information Strategy for the Modern NHS 1998-2005. A National Strategy for Local Implementation.* London: NHSE.
NHSE (National Health Service Executive) (1998a) *Clinical Effectiveness Indicators: A Consultation Document.* London: DoH.
NHSE (National Health Service Executive) (1998b) *National Framework for Assessing Performance.* London: NHSE.
NHSE (National Health Service Executive) (1998c) *Clinical Governance Moving from Rhetoric to Reality.* London: NHSE.
NHSE (National Health Service Executive) (1999) *Learning To Manage Health Information.* London: NHSE.
National Health Service Information Authority (1999a) *Reviewing Health Information Services: ETD Support for LIS Development.* Bristol: NHS Information Authority.
National Health Service Information Authority (1999b) *Assessing the Impact of LIS on IM&T: ETD Support for LIS Development.* Bristol: NHS Information Authority.
National Health Service Information Authority (1999c) *Training Needs Analysis: ETD Support for LIS Development.*
NHSME (National Health Service Management Executive) (1991) *Junior Doctors: The New Deal.* London: NHSME.
NHSME (National Health Service Management Executive) (1993) *Nursing in Primary Health Care – New World, New Opportunities.* Leeds: NHSME.
Neubauer, J. (1997) Beyond hierarchy: working on the edge of chaos [editorial]. *Journal of Nursing Management* 5: 65–7.
New Zealand Guidelines Group. Accessed 21-11-1999 http://www.nzgg.org.nz/index.htm.
'NT' Learning Curve (1997) Clinical guidelines – developing clinical guidelines. *NT Learning Curve* 1(1): 10–11.
Nursing Standard (1996) Ten steps to producing clinical guidelines. *Nursing Standard* 10(32): 32.
O'Donnell, M. (1993) How to enable staff to empower patients. *Nursing Standard* 8(12): 38–9.
Ogbonna, E. (1991) Managing organisational culture: fantasy or reality? *Human Resource Management Journal* 3(2): 42–54.
Osbourne, P. (1991) Research in nurse education. In Cormack, D.F.S. (ed.) *The Research Process in Nursing.* Oxford: Blackwell Scientific.
Pearson, A. (1989) Therapeutic nursing – transforming roles and theories in actions. *Recent Advances in Nursing* 24: 123–51.

Pearson, A. (1998) Excellence in care: future dimensions for effective nursing. *Nursing Times Research* **3**(1): 25–7.

Pearson, M. (2000) Making a difference through research: how can nurses turn the vision into reality? [guest editorial]. *Nursing Times Research* **5**(2): 85–6.

Peplau, H. (1969) Professional closeness: a special kind of involvement with patient, client and family. *Nursing Forum* **4**: 342–60.

Perske, R. (1972) Cited in Baldwin, S. (1999) Care in the community for people with a learning disability: choice, opportunity and risk. *Mental Healthcare* **2**(5): 167–9.

Pontin, D. (1999) Primary nursing. *Journal of Advanced Nursing* **29**(3): 584–91.

Proctor, B. (1992) Maps and models of supervision. In Hawkins, P. and Shohet, R. (eds) *Supervision in the Helping Professions*. Milton Keynes: Open University Press.

Rafferty, A. M. and Traynor, M. (1999) The research-practice gap in nursing: lessons from the research policy debate. *Nursing Times Research* **4**(6): 458–65.

Rappolt, S.G. (1997) Clinical guidelines and the fate of medical autonomy in Ontario. *Social Science and Medicine* **44**(7): 977–87.

Read, S. (1991) Case study of management changes in the NHS. *Nursing Times* **87**(16 January): 53.

Read, S. (1999) Nurse-led care: the importance of management support. *Nursing Times Research* **4**(6): 408–21.

Redfern, S., Normand, C., Christian, S., Gilmore, A., Murrells, T., Norman, I. and Stevens, W. (1997) An evaluation of nursing development units. *Nursing Times Research* **2**(4): 292–302.

Robinson, J. (1992) Introduction: Beginning the study of nursing policy. In Robinson, J., Gray, A. and Elkan, R. (eds) *Policy Issues in Nursing*. Milton Keynes: Open University Press.

Rolfe, G. (1996) *Closing the Theory–Practice Gap. A New Paradigm for Nursing*. Oxford: Butterworth Heinemann.

Rolfe, G. (1998) The theory–practice gap in nursing: from research-based practice to practitioner based research. *Journal of Advanced Nursing* **28**(3): 672–9.

Rosenburg, W. and Donald, A. (1995) Evidence-based medicine; an approach to clinical problem solving. *British Medical Journal* **310**: 1122–6.

Rosswurm, M.A. and Larrabee, J.H. (1999) A model for change to evidence based practice. *Image: Journal of Nursing Scholarship* **31**(4): 317–22.

Rotter, J.B. (1966) Generalised expectations for internal versus external control of reinforcement: a major variable in behaviour therapy. *Psychological Monographs* **80**(1).

RCN (Royal College of Nursing) (1998a) *Evidence to the Pay Review Body for 1999.* London: RCN.

RCN (Royal College of Nursing) (1998b) *Edlines.* London: RCN.

RCN (Royal College of Nursing) (1999a) *Clinical Guidelines: What You Need To Know.* London: RCN.

Royal College of Nursing (1999b) *Clinical Guidelines: Involving Patients and Service Users.* London: RCN.

Rumbold, G. (1986) *Ethics in Nursing Practice.* London: Baillière Tindall.

Sackett, D. and Rosenberg, W. (1995) On the need for evidence-based medicine. *Auditorium* **2**: 3–7.

Sackett, D.L., Rosenberg, W., Gray, J.A.M., Haynes, R.B. and Richardson, W.S. (1996) Evidence based medicine: what it is and what it isn't. *British Medical Journal* **312**: 71–2.

Saha, A. (1995) Clinical guidelines [letter, comment]. *British Medical Journal* **310**(6980): 670.

Salvage, J. (1992). The new nursing: empowering patients or empowering nurses? In Robinson, J., Gray, A. and Elkan, R. (eds) *Policy Issues in Nursing.* Milton Keynes: Open University Press.

Salvage, J. (1998) Evidence based practice: a mixture of motives? *Nursing Times Research* **3**(6): 406–18.

Saunders, P. (1995) Encouraging patients to take part in their own care. *Nursing Times* **91**(9): 42–43.

Savage, J. (1990) The theory and practice of the 'new nursing'. Occasional paper. *Nursing Times* **86**(1): 42–5.

Scally, P. and Donaldson, L. (1998) Clinical governance and the drive for quality improvement in the new NHS in England. *British Medical Journal* **317**: 61–5.

ScHARR (School of Health and Related Research) (1997) *The New Government's Health Agenda.* Sheffield: KPMG.

Scott, I. (1999) An opportunity for nurses to influence the future of healthcare development. *Nursing Times Research* **4**(3): 170–5.

Scottish Intercollegiate Guidelines Network (1997) *Implementation of the St Vincent Declaration. The Care of Diabetic Patients in Scotland. Management of Diabetic Foot Disease: A National Clinical Guideline Recommended for Use in Scotland.* Edinburgh: SIGN.

Scottish Intercollegiate Guidelines Network. Accessed 12-10-2000 http://www/show.scot.nhs.uk/sign/.

Seers, K. and Milne, R. (1997) Randomised controlled trials in nursing [editorial]. *Quality in Healthcare* **6**(1): 1.

Shekelle, P.G., Woolf, S.H., Eccles, M. and Grimshaw, J. (1999) Clinical guidelines: developing guidelines. *British Medical Journal* **318**(7183): 593–6.

Smith Blancett, S. and Flarey, D. (1995) *Reengineering Nursing and Healthcare.* Maryland: Aspen Publishers.

180   *References*

Smith, C.E., Buck, S., Colligan, E., Derndt, P. and Sollie, T. (1980) Differences in importance ratings of self-care geriatric patients and the nurses who care for them. *International Journal of Nursing Studies* **17**(3): 145–53.

Stevens, J. (1997) Improving integration between research and practice as a means of developing evidence based healthcare. *Nursing Times Research* **2**(1): 7–15.

Styles, M.M. (1982) *On Nursing Toward a New Endowment.* St Louis: C.V. Mosby.

Summerton, H. (2000) Who cares? *Nursing Times* **96**(1): 30–1.

Tait, T. (1999) *Doubly Disadvantaged? The Challenge for the New Decade.* London: RCN.

Taylor, B. (1996) Parent as partners in care. *Paediatric Nursing* **8**(4): 24–7.

Teasdale, K. (1987) Partnership with patients. *Professional Nurse* **2**(12): 17–19.

Thomas, L.H., McColl, E., Cullum, N., Rousseau, N. and Soutter, J. (1999) Clinical guidelines in nursing, midwifery and the therapies: a systematic review. *Journal of Advanced Nursing* **30**(1): 40–50.

Thomson, R., Lavender, M. and Madhok, R. (1995) How to ensure that guidelines are effective. *British Medical Journal* **311**: 237–42.

Tierney, A. (1998) The politics of the NHS R&D agenda. *Nursing Times Research* **3**(6): 419–20.

Tschudin, V. (1989) Informed consent. *Surgical Nurse* **12**(6): 15–17.

Twigg, J. and Atkin, K. (1994) *Carers Perceived: Policy and Practice in Informed Care.* Milton Keynes: Open University Press.

UKCC (United Kingdom Central Council for Nursing, Midwifery and Health Visiting) (1992a) *The Scope of Professional Practice.* London: UKCC.

UKCC (United Kingdom Central Council for Nursing, Midwifery and Health Visiting) (1992b) *Code of Professional Conduct for the Nurse, Midwife and Health Visitor.* London: UKCC.

UKCC (United Kingdom Central Council for Nursing, Midwifery and Health Visiting) (1994) *The Future of Professional Practice. The Council's Standards for Education and Practice Following Registration.* London: UKCC.

UKCC (United Kingdom Central Council for Nursing, Midwifery and Health Visiting) (1996) *Position Statement on Clinical Supervision for Nursing and Health Visiting.* London: UKCC.

UKCC (United Kingdom Central Council for Nursing, Midwifery and Health Visiting) (1998) *Paper to Inform Developments of the Specialist Practice Framework: The Assessment of Competence.* London: UKCC.

UKCC (United Kingdom Central Council for Nursing, Midwifery and Health Visiting) (1999a) *Fitness for Practice.* The UKCC

Commission for Nursing and Midwifery Education (chairman Sir Leonard Peach). London: UKCC.

UKCC (United Kingdom Central Council for Nursing, Midwifery and Health Visiting) (1999b) *Nursing in Secure Environments.* London: UKCC.

Veeramah, V. (1995) A study to identify the attitudes and needs of qualified staff concerning the use of research findings in clinical practice within mental health settings. *Journal of Advanced Nursing* **22**: 855–61.

Wade, S. (1995) Partnership in care: a critical review. *Nursing Standard* **9**(48): 333–5.

Walczak, J.R., MacGuire, D.B. and Haisfield, M.G. (1994) A survey of research related activities and perceived barriers to research utilisation among professional oncology nurses. *Oncology Nursing Forum* **21**(4): 710–15.

Walsh, M.P. (1998) What is evidence? A critical view for nursing. *Clinical Effectiveness in Nursing* **2**: 86–93.

Walshe, K., Ham, C. and Appleby, J. (1995) Given in evidence. *Health Service Journal* **29**(June): 28–9.

Waterworth, S. and Luker, K. A. (1990) Reluctant collaborators: do patients want to be involved in decisions concerning care? *Journal of Advanced Nursing* **15**: 971–6.

Webb, C (1986) *Feminist Practice in Women's Healthcare.* Chichester: John Wiley & Sons.

Webb, C. (1996) Action research. In Cormack, D.F.S. (ed.) *The Research Process in Nursing.* Oxford: Blackwell Scientific.

Webster, C. (1998) *The Health Services Since the War.* London: HMSO.

West, E. and Newton, J. (1997) Clinical guidelines [editorial]. *British Medical Journal* **315**(7104): 324.

West, M. (1999) Communication and team working in healthcare. *Nursing Times Research* **4**(1): 8–17.

West, M.A. and Poulton, B.C. (1997) A failure of function. Teamwork in primary healthcare. *Journal of Interprofessional Care* **11**(2): 205–16.

Wheeler, C.E. and Chinn, P. (1991) *Peace and Power. A Handbook of Feminist Process,* 3rd edn. Buffalo: Margaret Daughters.

White, S.J. (1997) Evidence based practice and nursing: the new panacea? *British Journal of Nursing* **6**: 175–8.

Williams, J.G. (1999) Guidelines for clinical guidelines should distinguish between national and local production [letter, comment]. *British Medical Journal* **318**(7188): 942.

Wilson, J. (1997) An introduction to multidisciplinary pathways of care. Unpublished document.

Wilson-Barnett, J. and Fordham, M. (1982) *Recovery from Illness*. Chichester: John Wiley & Sons.

Winstanley, J. (1999) *Methods for Evaluating the Effectiveness of Clinical Supervision*. Clinical Monograph. London: Nursing Times Books.

Woolf, S.H., Grol, R., Hutchinson, A., Eccles, M. and Grimshaw, J. (1999) Clinical guidelines: potential benefits, limitations, and harms of clinical guidelines. *British Medical Journal* **318**(7182): 527–30.

Yorkshire Regional Health Authority (1991) *Developing the Research Resource in Nursing and the Therapy Professions*. Harrogate: YRHA.

Index